What is eczema?

A path to ending the misery

2nd Edition

What is eczema?

A path to ending the misery

2nd Edition

Dr Harley Farmer

PhD BVSc(Hons) BVBiol(Path) MRCVS

Foreword by Professor Terence J Ryan

Second edition first published in 2016. The first edition was published in 2015
© Dr Harley Farmer

Registered office of publisher:
NewGenn Ltd, 4 Hereward Way Business Park, Harling Road, Roudham, Norfolk, NR16 2SR, United Kingdom.

For information about how to apply for permission to reuse the copyright material in this book and for customer services please see our website www.newgenn.com

Library of Congress Cataloging-in-Publication Data

Farmer, Harley.
      What is eczema? A path to ending the misery. 2nd Edition.
      ISBN 978-0-9569707-3-2

A catalogue record of this book is available from the British Library.

Front cover photography: Waterfall Walk, County Donegal, Ireland. © 2014 Dr Anne-Marie Farmer; all rights reserved.

Set in Bookman by Ian Taylor - www.taylorthorneprint.co.uk

Printed in Great Britain by Taylor Thorne Print Ltd, UK

Harley Farmer in this cornucopia of a text calls himself Philosopher, Romantic and Eternal Optimist. He has a veterinary background without requiring much chat to patients, but here after many hours of reading about atopic eczema in humans, he spends much time in conversation with patients and their exasperated parents. One learns what atopic eczema is like as an experience. His final sentence is "As always, the outcome for patients will rest on the skills, knowledge, perspective and training of the person responsible for their care". This indisputable statement would be a good beginning.

His most valuable contribution is perhaps the simple argument that loss of the skin's barrier function provides entry points to deeper epidermis and dermis thereby testing the skin's immunosurveillance system triggering of an inflammatory reaction to foreign agents including those prescribed. Such a reaction is designed to be helpful but some of the foreign agents such as emollients which do good on the anaerobic surface may not be so well appreciated by much deeper healthy living cells.

Harley is marketing his products which are harmless and a substitute for many therapeutic agents that can have adverse effects. I do not feel confident that my profession has mastered management of eczema nor that its prescribing habits never do any harm.

I am confident that Harley's approach is harmless and that his successes will be numerous.

These exerts come from EXeczema® successes you will find in this book. They want you to know eczema can be beaten and kept away. Their success is living proof.

"I have subsequently recommended Dr Harley to friends, whose children have varying forms of eczema and I cannot thank him enough for making the process so easy and successful". **Phili Wilson, Wiltshire, England**

"He easily builds good bonds with children and Max liked him immediately ... We look forward to our lives without eczema and a new lifelong friendship". **Jill Wildish, England**

"To any parent who has a child with eczema I would definitely recommend they try it but not before reading the book because they will not give their 100% commitment as they won't understand the program". **Nicki Rooprai, UK**

"... more than year since the eczema disappeared and never came back. ... his own immunity was supported and not pushed down by strong chemicals. Many thanks to Dr Harley Farmer". **Josef Toth, Unken, Austria**

"I am so glad that my eczema has gone and I can have long nails and not have to worry about people laughing at me and now the things I enjoy are more enjoyable". **Beeka Hindle, Norfolk, England**

"Having suffered with painful, debilitating and persistent hand eczema for over 25 years, I thought I would never be free from this horrible condition. ... I have healthy new skin on my hands and the difference this has made to my life is enormous". **Susan Ellis, Cambridge, England**

"The legs and feet look great! They are not fiery or itchy. We are no longer getting the breakouts. In fact, the eczema has GONE! ... She is now 94". **Joan Flint, Queensland, Australia**

CHAPTER 1

The incredible journey made credible

There are many people saying "**we can't**" cure eczema. There are a lot more saying "**we did**".

How can the two groups coexist in this time of instant global communication? Perhaps my personal story will provide an answer. As a young man at university I had bad eczema on my face and chest. It went on for years, was painful, embarrassing and a social inconvenience. At the time I felt fortunate in having friends who were medical students giving me personal tuition in the fact that eczema can't be cured. They were very sorry and very adamant; I had an incurable disease and all they could do was help me manage it. I knew their advice was based on evidence-based medical research and they genuinely believed what they were saying.

That was pretty depressing stuff. As it happens I'm a perpetual optimist so I politely accepted their assistance and set out on a personal journey to understand eczema. To cut a multi-decade story short I came to realise those who say "we can't" and those who say "we did" were only separated by a point of view; a play on words.

The eczema-can't-be-cured group were really emphasising the point that "**we** can't" cure it. The other group had trouble understanding that viewpoint as they had ended their eczema and it had never returned. To them eczema had ceased to be a topic so they had little reason to debate the word cure. They lived in the *time after* eczema. That's where I've spent my last 40 years.

I've become what one of my friends jokingly called a "multi-ologist" because I developed a degree of expertise in immunology, pathology, dermatology, psychology, bacteriology, virology and more. In essence I'm an *-ology junkie*! I just love collecting useful bits of information and storing them away for future use.

Someone with that sort of mind becomes unemployable so I created my own companies to do my own thing. To me there is a lot of human suffering which simply fails to make sense and eczema was a common example. The medical view was "we can't" cure eczema and they based their view on medical facts. Yet I could see another fact. The vast majority of people who ever developed eczema grew out of it and never suffered from it again. They are the ones who say "we did" cure eczema. I had an empathy with both groups; in my -ology searches I studied the medical literature and saw their facts, yet I had cured my eczema and was therefore in that very large group who could say "we did".

I strongly believe the answers are out there and my skill lies in finding the right questions. What kept the minority in eczema? What kept it going in one child when it disappeared permanently for most of their friends? Why are both the "we can't" and "we did" groups correct?

It's easiest to begin with the "we can't" group as the facts are irrefutable. These folk seem to view eczema as a disease and quite logically use drugs to overcome the disease. Using steroids to manage eczema is a good example. Yet there is a problem. When you delve deep into their medical evidence you find the fact that steroids reduce ceramide production by keratinocytes reducing lipid bilayers and preventing the formation of optimal skin barrier. Don't panic — I won't stay in this medical jargon for long. This evidence simply means steroids help make skin porous allowing foreign chemicals to penetrate inducing inflammation. That is eczema.

Some of the people who prescribe topical steroids for eczema may be alarmed when I make such a powerful statement in this book written for the general public. I refer such people to the review of medical literature in the back of this book and ask them whether they have confidence in their own evidence. The peer-reviewed articles I'm quoting are listed there and the evidence of the negative effect of steroids on skin is available for all to see. It has been for years.

Another evidence-based fact is that mineral oils penetrate a sub-optimal skin barrier becoming lodged in and disrupting the ceramide bi-layers making the skin barrier more porous allowing the penetration of foreign chemicals which induce inflammation.

That is eczema. Mineral oil is a component in most moisturisers, emollients, creams and ointments; the very products suggested for use with eczema. Again I refer anyone who is upset by this revelation to the relevant peer-reviewed article in the appendix. That evidence has been known for years yet the products are still recommended.

The drugs most commonly used to manage eczema contain mineral oil and/or steroids. It can be argued that both maintain eczema. Is that why those who say "we can't" cure eczema are right? If the products they favour to *manage* eczema actually *maintain* eczema they will certainly be right.

May I please make a heart-felt plea at this early stage? Would anyone who is apoplectic over the previous paragraphs please examine ALL the evidence-based peer-reviewed articles listed in the literature review in the appendix at the back of the book. If that evidence is wrong then my premise is wrong and I will change it. If that evidence is right then I will continue to present my views in this way for the benefit of those who suffer from eczema. All this information is available to those members of the general public who take the time to find it; I am simply making it available for those who lack that time.

This information will also make life much easier for doctors who feel they currently spend too much of their valuable time seeing eczema patients time and time again. If those doctors had reason to move on from the "we can't" viewpoint they will have an ever increasing number of patients who say "we did". A major objective of this book is to show doctors why that transition is valid and based on their own published peer-reviewed evidence. The public like to believe their doctors act on medical evidence and this book seeks to translate that evidence into the common vernacular. Eczema is an issue for both doctors and patients and wonderful things happen when I lead doctors and patients to work together with a positive perspective.

Why are those who say "we did" so positive? Mainly because they view eczema as an imbalance. If it's not a disease no drug or cure is needed; just regain balance and the skin will fix itself.

At this point I know I'm at serious risk of some people feeling I'm belittling their suffering. Please remember that I have suffered from bad eczema and I have witnessed the terrible suffering the burden of eczema has heaped upon families. When I use the word imbalance please appreciate that I know an imbalance can be severe. Also please be very aware that I know drugs must be used when severe eczema induces conditions like life-threatening septicaemia. However once the acute issue is addressed the choice is to maintain eczema or end it. Both choices are available depending how you wish to utilise the same cache of evidence. That evidence means having eczema or not is a matter of choice; the choice of whether you want to be in the "we can't" or "we did" group. The evidence is the same; how you use that evidence dictates the outcome.

The imbalance leading to eczema involves a lot more than just skin. I have found it wise to provide broad-based coaching to help people who are ready to end eczema. The main text of this book reflects the coaching methods which have worked best, so there is a degree of intentional repetition and many questions designed to focus the mind on specific points. Even though the main text is written for the general public, doctors and eczema specialists can obviously read it so they know what those they are serving have learned. There are also occasional places where the subject of the text is directed specifically to the advisers.

In contrast, the review of the medical literature in the appendix at the end of the book is written for those with medical qualifications or specialist training in eczema. It is presented in the technical jargon utilised in the medical and scientific literature. It's the peer-reviewed, evidence-based, research on which best medical practice evolves. It can still be read by members of the general public who want to learn what evidence is available to those advising on eczema.

The book is intended to be inclusive and you can expect regular revisions of the text in subsequent editions with updates on the medical literature. Eczema is evolving quickly in reflection of other changes in society and this book will progress and evolve in a similar fashion.

When conducting one-to-one personal coaching, a good coach will utilise the language patterns of the individual being helped so the person appreciates they are the focus of attention. That presents a challenge for an author who wants all the readers to feel they, as individuals, are the focus. To make it truly inclusive, a variety of language patterns are intermingled here to repeatedly remind every reader they are the intended focus.

At regular intervals you will find stories of people who have ended their eczema and thereafter kept their skin in happy balance. Some of them progressed to normal healthy skin in a matter of weeks and others took longer. When properly utilised, the clues presented in this book will allow eczema-prone skin to heal itself. I want to stress at the outset that it is the **knowledge** and the **action** to implement it which lead to the success. The very gentle skin cleansing products I provide will never do the job alone as they are simply too gentle to break through the damage certain skincare products cause. The successes range in age from a few months to over 90 years and are a representative sample of those who have completed the EXeczema® programme. They share their stories here so others around the world can benefit.

Eczema has been plaguing people for a very long time, providing ample opportunity for those in authority to agree on a definition. The definitions presented below were those available in May 2014.

The definition in the Oxford Concise Medical Dictionary is

> "**eczema** *n.* a common itchy skin disease characterised by reddening (erythema) and vesicle formation, which may lead to weeping and crusting. It is endogenous, or constitutional, i.e. outside agents do not play a primary role (*compare* DERMATITIS), but in some contexts the terms 'dermatitis' and 'eczema' are used interchangeably".

The American Academy of Dermatology website says

> "Eczema is a general term. Dermatologists use it to describe skin conditions that can cause the skin to swell and discolor. The skin is often dry and itchy. Sometimes blisters form. The most common type of eczema is atopic dermatitis. When people say "eczema," this is often what they mean — but not always." www.aad.org

Those two are written for mainly medical audiences making it worth looking at others intended for the general public.

If you search for 'eczema' in Wikipedia you'll see

"Dermatitis or eczema is inflammation of the skin. ... The term eczema is also commonly used to describe atopic dermatitis or atopic eczema. In some languages dermatitis and eczema are synonymous, while in other languages dermatitis implies an acute condition and eczema a chronic one".

The website of the National Eczema Society in Britain has a statement that

"Eczema (also known as dermatitis) is a dry skin condition which is highly individual in its nature". They go on to say "Atopic eczema is a genetic condition based on the interaction between a number of genes and environmental factors. In most cases there will be a family history of either eczema or one of the other 'atopic' conditions i.e asthma or hay fever". www.eczema.org

The American National Eczema Association's website says

"Eczema is a general term for any type of dermatitis or "inflammation of the skin". They also say "Atopic Dermatitis (which is often called eczema) is an itchy, red rash." www.nationaleczema.org

Are you confused yet? If you are, you're far from being alone. The condition has been around for ages yet there seems to be a lack of agreement. That adds an extra challenge to those fighting the condition, wouldn't you agree?

Those are 'working level' definitions and adding another at that level is very unlikely to help. So I offer one at a higher level.

Eczema is a state of confusion about red skin.

How can a new definition at another level be helpful? In a number of ways.

People who favour the working-level definitions justifiably agree my mention of "red skin" is too simplistic. It's too broad. Why would I want to create a unified objection to my definition? Because there would finally be something for all the other definition providers to agree on. People who agree are more likely to make progress.

Notice how my definition contains two elements. The first is that eczema is a *state* of confusion. To that, you could expect universal agreement and discussion in which everyone's opinion is welcome and everyone can take part. That's being inclusive.

Much of the scientific and medical debate is in technical jargon the general public is not expected to understand. I read the scientific and medical articles because I'm comfortable with what profilaggrin is, why inadequate FLG expression is so relevant to eczema, how a lack of urocanic acid in the *stratum corneum* is important and why lowered or raised levels of IgE are useful indicators.

For readers who want an up to date summary of the technical medical literature, I have provided that in the appendix at the end of this book. It is included for two reasons:

1. so anyone, medical or otherwise, can read it and know they are up to date for the time this edition of the book was written, and
2. so anyone with technical and medical expertise who might be considering lazy negative criticism of what I present in this book can know my views are based on *their* most current evidence-based research.

The technical literature offers many clues on the finer details of what is happening in eczema, yet it adds to the confusion by its sheer massive volume. Therefore I would like to take this early opportunity to set the tone for the rest of the book.

I once had a wise and highly experienced professor teach me that "there is **art** and **science** in medicine and the art lies in knowing when NOT to use the science". He was saying that both have a key role and patients are served best when art and science are in balance. He was referring to what is often called 'bedside manner', something many people would like to see more of in modern medicine. With the deluge of technical data now being generated on so many diseases, it has become necessary for doctors to concentrate very hard on alleviating individual specific symptoms. Time is precious and they may have little of it left to develop and practice their skills in the art of balancing the whole patient.

In the specific field of eczema, how often do doctors prescribe steroids to alleviate the single symptom of skin inflammation without finding time to consider the whole patient? The skin inflammation is important, especially in severe eczema, but it's only one of many symptoms, each of which is providing helpful clues. If they concentrate too much of their efforts on that one symptom, might they forgo opportunities to help the whole patient? When this extends to most of the medical profession, it becomes standard practice to 'manage' the disease by alleviating one symptom. They become very good at ending skin inflammation and have little reason to think about ending eczema. Their utilisation of art and science can lead to imbalance within the patient.

In one respect that's a little unfair as most of the effort in managing eczema actually involves the use of moisturizers to overcome dry skin. So let's look at dry skin as another single symptom. What is gained by placing a lot of effort into managing dry skin with moisturizers? That's an easy one to answer; the skin feels less dry. Good. Again, excellent progress has been made in addressing one symptom of eczema.

But do the patients feel that has cured their eczema? Very unlikely, for two reasons:

1. they've been told repeatedly that eczema can't be cured so why should they expect moisturisers to provide such an unexpected outcome, and
2. the moisturiser was only ever intended to end one specific symptom, not the entire disease.

That has led to the established official view that "eczema can't be cured". Have you ever heard that? Or said it yourself? If you can't cure it, it's best to manage it, correct?

Are you pleased to see such an exclusive and divisive choice? You EITHER manage it OR cure it, but you can't have both. To manage it you concentrate on ending the main symptoms with moisturizers and steroids.

At this point we now have the two symptoms of dry skin and skin inflammation being considered. At the risk of being repetitive, does the patient who has been 'managed' in this limited way feel their eczema has been cured? No, for the same two reasons; they believe it when people they trust say it can't be cured and the two treatments were only intended to end two symptoms.

Have we even considered the whole patient yet? No. There is a lot more to that person than patches of dry reddened skin. Does the belief that eczema can't be cured reside in the skin or in the mind? It's in the mind, isn't it? When doctors tell a patient "eczema can't be cured", are they speaking to the person's skin or their mind? This is approaching the point of being silly, yet would you agree it helps distinguish between the symptoms and the person?

This might look like an improvement as we now have three aspects of the person being involved in the management of eczema:

1. moisturisers to manage the dry skin,
2. steroids to manage the inflamed skin,
3. advice that eczema can't be cured to manage expectations.

Most patients willingly use the moisturisers, begrudgingly accept the steroids and hear the advice that eczema can't be cured. After all, they want to trust their doctor and all three aspects of the management are emanating from that source. If they check on the internet they'll find patients are being managed the same way all around the developed world. If it's global it must be right!

All that raises an important question. Why would anyone want to continue reading this book if the skin and mind of eczema patients are being so well managed?

If you have no reasonable answer to that question, I implore you to put this book aside. It would most likely just annoy you. If you have eczema or are helping someone with eczema, it might even elevate your stress levels and worsen the eczema. Put the book aside; you have enough to worry about.

However, if your answer ventures towards valuing the whole patient or a desire to achieve balance then please read on. This book encompasses both the art and science taking every opportunity to balance them and end the eczema. You will soon learn why eczema *is being cured* every day.

Throughout this book you will find key aspects of the known science integrated into the text in a readable format. The science is the most up to date I could find in the Addenbrooke's Hospital medical library in Cambridge, England. That science is expanding all the time and I find it's becoming more and more complicated. I'm repeatedly humbled by the incredible diversity of the immune markers experts can find within the skin and blood of eczema sufferers. Sadly the researchers repeatedly say it's still impossible to determine whether the immune markers are the cause of eczema or the result of eczema. If you haven't detected it already, you will come to realise I'm an eternal optimist and I'll continue finding time to avidly read their wonderful articles.

All that complexity and resultant confusion has its place, but someone associated with eczema only needs to see red skin to know something is out of balance. The experts will continue providing excellent science and remain confused. Fascinated and enthralled, but confused.

In this book I dispel that confusion while presenting the more helpful aspects of the most up to date science.

A second way my higher-level definition of eczema helps is to legitimise the state of confusion. Why? Because it allows all those who are confused over eczema to realise that's the best choice when the information available is so confusing. I've seen high levels of confusion among medical experts and the public, in equal measures.

This universal confusion is a good thing as it demonstrates how the way we have been looking at eczema fails to serve the sufferers well. I ask people to accept the confusion and applaud it. All those examining eczema in the conventional way share that confusion.

So relax, you're doing as well as the rest of them. Your **confusion** is justified.

The challenge comes when someone like me, a PhD, a philosopher and lifelong thinker, takes the time to look at eczema from a different perspective and suggest **clarity**.

What induced me to allocate all that precious time? Very simply, it was mothers thanking me for "curing" the eczema in their children. You will better appreciate my initial confusion when you realise I was not working with children at the time and I didn't know any of the mothers!

There was something wonderful going on and I had absolutely no idea what it was — even though I was apparently causing it! Ample grounds for confusion, wouldn't you agree?

What does a romantic optimist like me do in such a situation? Investigate. I'd had bad eczema as a young man, rid myself of it and learned from the experience. Could I have subconsciously and inadvertently included that knowledge into something else I was doing? The answer was yes. At the time my work related to reducing infections in hospitals and the hand hygiene products I'd helped develop were alleviating the dermatitis so often seen on the hands of nurses. These were the products being used on the children when their eczema disappeared.

Having rid myself of eczema and then progressed through a career of successfully ending other diseases, I was well placed to see the events in these children from a different perspective. I hasten to add that each and every one of them may have been a coincidence where the child was about to end the eczema anyway. It's a well established fact that the vast majority of children 'grow out of eczema' and the safest presumption was that all those children just happened to be ending their eczema at the time my products were used on their skin. I knew and fully appreciated that.

But since I was not actually working with the children or their mothers, I was free to wonder if something other than coincidence was behind what appeared to be such good news.

I chose to ask a question. What products had been used on the children's damaged skin before my products were introduced? The ingredient lists from almost all those previously-used products caused me great alarm! If those ingredients were detected by the immune system, there **would** be inflammation as the immune system tried to protect the children from the foreign chemicals. That induced me to ask a question which only had one answer; a very scary answer.

Could the products used to *manage* eczema actually *maintain* eczema?

The answer was yes. They could.

However, as we all know, saying they COULD be involved is a very long way from showing they ARE involved. You can reach that conclusion without a PhD; without delving into the murky depths of philosophy.

This is a good time to appreciate why a person in my position is wise to remain very quiet when you first generate a question with such far reaching ramifications. Many millions of people are entangled in eczema and it's very unwise to destabilise millions of people. Experience suggests it's likely this question or something like it had been raised before yet I could not find an answer mentioned anywhere.

That presented me with choices. I could:

- say "what a wonderful question" and proceed to ignore it,
- stop what I was doing and focus entirely on this seemingly very important question, or
- do a bit of both; continue the other infection prevention work I was doing while I carefully tip-toed around the edges of the minefield this explosive question represented.

I chose the third. First, I dug deep into my philosopher's toolkit to find weaknesses in ideas that formed around the question. As expected, weaknesses did arise. However, when each of those was overcome, the fundamental question became more relevant. Each time, the answer became a stronger yes.

One option I'm glad to say was not available to me was to use those products on a healthy child to cause eczema. I would never harm a child; yet I could do that on myself. I had been free of eczema for decades but application of those products brought my eczema back. When I stopped applying the products, my skin healed itself and the eczema went away.

I'm a PhD, a Doctor of Philosophy, and I love my science. However, that rigorous training teaches you to go much deeper than a simple experiment on yourself, even if it is repeated and gives the same results every time. There was still a long way to go.

I would never want to cause eczema in children so my other

option was to *end* eczema in children. Each success would have to be viewed as a possible coincidence of eczema leaving just when I arrived, but enough happy coincidences would evolve into a worthwhile story.

That's what happened. Friends of mine whose children had eczema learned of my question and opted to do what the original mothers had done. They stopped using the products. The result was a pleasing number of children who developed perfect skin and could move on from eczema. A few other children developed perfect looking skin but still had very itchy skin, and a tiny minority of those opted to continue habitually scratching certain patches of skin.

Yet overall, the pattern of positive outcomes made further investigation an attractive choice. This book sets out my current thinking on how eczema begins, what keeps it going, how to end it and how to prevent it coming back.

What I'm offering is KNOWLEDGE. Without that knowledge, the eczema continues or comes back as the dreaded 'flare-ups'.

This is a good-news story with a happy ending and like any good story, the happy ending only offers true value when you read the whole story. I ask you to read all the way through from beginning to end. The really technical part is in the appendix; it does not need to clutter our good story. Assuming of course, that the story teller has taken the 'scary technical bits' and woven them into the story line. Trust me; they're there. Just relax and have fun finding them, if that's what you call fun.

In chapter 12 you will find some questions I pose regarding the current paradigms underpinning the treatment and management of eczema, especially atopic eczema in children. Those questions only have relevance within the whole story. The questions have been examined by some highly influential medical individuals who've found them very intriguing, and intensely challenging.

Eczema relates to many people:

- those like me who have moved on from it and gained control,
- sufferers who still have eczema,
- family members who are helping those with eczema,
- researchers who provide the wonderful new clues, and
- medical people who want the best for their patients.

The key theme of this book is inclusion so all of us can contribute to improving health and happiness.

Now, let's return to the many definitions of eczema, all of which have validity. And they all add to the confusion. Let's all agree to see that confusion. That provides control, something I find most people associated with eczema crave.

EXeczema® Success

Henry Toth - a remarkable story

Henry was an extreme case. Only half year old baby when first flair up came. His skin was burning all over his head and we ended up in hospital with wet eczema all over his body. Strong steroids cure followed and he was getting better, but

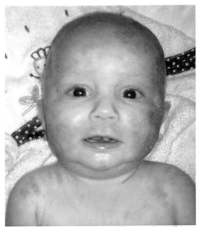

another two strong flair ups came within two weeks and his eczema was constantly active. Red spots all over his body, blistery, first getting wet and building thick yellow crust afterwards. No cute baby skin at all.

It was very distressing for us parents to see our baby struggle so much. We had to wrap him up every night to prevent him scratching himself and be constantly around him. We had to sleep with him at night to hold his hand and legs to avoid scratching. Any time when he freed himself he hurt himself very badly and scratched until he bled. It was definitely serious and a very stressful time. But the biggest problem was that we did not want to use strong chemicals on the skin for such a little baby. And this is the most important fact on NewGenn for parents. We were searching very hard to find the right way to get it under control without making any harm. We were coincidently introduced to Dr. Farmer and his methods and we had no other option, just trust him.

Skin was calming down first weeks and no erupting that hard anymore. It was two months of taking everyday photos and e-mailing them to UK to Dr. Farmer. Supported by Harley s every day advices we saw that disease disappearing step by step and that Henry s immunity is getting stronger to fight with his skin disease. Most helpful were NewGenn wipes which cleans the skin in a very gentle way. Very smart, perfectly working.

We will never forgot the first night he slept alone hands free, or when he slept on his belly or just the first days without gloves, even if we rather want to forget this whole misery we have gone through.

In the beginning our local doctor's prognosis was very dramatic, saying that Henry will develop strong allergies and probably asthma too.

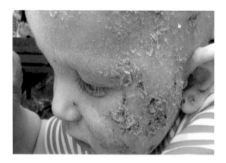 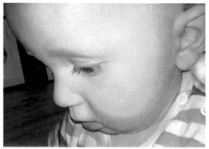

Now it is more than year since the eczema disappeared and never came back. And we know that our healthy baby is the result of the way he was cured and how his own immunity was supported and not pushed down by strong chemicals. It is one year since the eczema time and there is no trace of any skin disease, any allergy or asthma. Our Henry is just a happy healthy child.

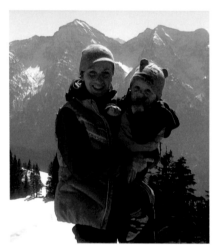

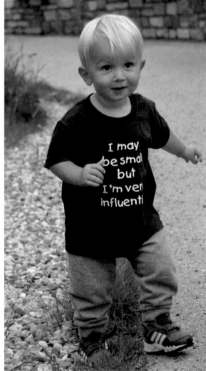

Many thanks to Dr. Harley Farmer.
Oct. 2014, Josef Toth,
Unken, Salzburg, Austria.

CHAPTER 2

Share the appreciation

To reach the happy ending of this journey, it's wise to know our starting place. My aim in writing this book is to create a mass awareness and understanding of eczema and show a way forward. I'm known as the "Listening Doctor" for the way I like to hear, and place great value in, each person's experience and comments. Everyone who has been kind enough to share their frustration, misery and success can take personal credit for the good news revealed. It would be impractical to list all those who've been good enough to share. Instead, I will mention what they've said. If you feel you have something new to add, you can contact me so our collective knowledge increases to be shared again in a subsequent edition of the book. The first edition only lasted six months before this second edition was needed because of new information and ideas.

When you feel included, you'll be more likely to take positive action, wouldn't you agree? You will become part of the winning team. The intention is to let readers know their experiences and feelings are normal in the bad state called eczema.

Many millions of people around the world are caught in what I call the **eczema trap**. This book provides choices allowing you to end the eczema. You will be in control, most likely for the first time. It's left to each and every person to take the necessary action when they have the new knowledge presented here. That's why sharing the collective experiences of so many people whose lives had once been tainted by the condition has such important and powerful relevance.

If a lot of what's shared in this chapter feels familiar to you, I welcome you to the growing tide of people moving toward that happy state I've named EXeczema®, the time *after eczema*.

In this chapter, quotation marks are used around statements I've heard people make, either direct to me or in groups. For example, "I've tried everything and nothing works". This is done so readers can associate better with those who've been in the bad place called eczema and are no longer there; people who have moved on and the imbalance has not returned. My aim is to have readers feel an association with those who've shared. Since the EXeczema successes have arisen from those who have shared, this is intended to provide inclusion for those who are still wanting to end eczema. Each of the EXeczema successes chose to do something different and it's well known that difference brings hope.

"They make me feel like a nuisance for always coming back with the same problem" is something I hear from many of those I've invited to express how they feel their medical team views them. "It seems their job is done once they've made the diagnosis and used the word eczema". From that moment, "all they want to do is manage it". One mother was particularly upset when she felt the doctor was saying "the fault lay with my child for developing the eczema".

"It's not explained by the doctor" is a common frustration, especially from those who've continued to seek a logical understanding of the process which leads to eczema. When they fail to receive a useful reply, they feel as if they're being "dismissed by the doctor". When they receive the same from a consultant dermatologist, they tend to believe the "whole system has given up on me".

Those comments obviously come from the viewpoint of patients; from adult eczema victims or from parents of children with eczema. This is the best time to share some of the comments I hear from my medical colleagues who "feel really frustrated at not being able to do more". One of the greatest concerns expressed is "all I can do is manage the condition". When I press them on how they explain the condition, I'm usually told "it's called atopic for a good reason; nobody knows why the inflammation is happening".

When those medical views are taken into account, it's hardly surprising when doctors don't explain something they don't actually understand.

This is why I say doctors are also victims of eczema. They don't have reddened, itchy, flaky skin but they are affected in other ways.

One told me "when I look at my patient list for the day, it hurts to see the name of an eczematous child I know I haven't been able to help". That doctor genuinely wants to deliver a better outcome for his patient but simply lacks what is needed to achieve success. Repeatedly seeing that child for the same eczema "wears heavily" on the inherent professional desire to see patients overcome medical problems.

Steroids tend to evoke highly emotional comments. Many parents have told me "I'm really worried about putting steroids on my child's skin". A lady who'd had eczema for 70 years had been applying steroids since they were first put into skin creams. "What else can I do?" she asked. "Without the steroids the itching drives me crazy so I just have to tolerate whatever damage the steroids are doing to my skin".

Conversely, I've had doctors say "I'm not keen on steroids but if we don't settle the eczema down the child may scratch holes in their skin and end up with septicaemia (blood poisoning)". As they point out to anyone who wants to listen, "eczema is a terrible nuisance whereas septicaemia can kill, very rapidly". As one doctor said "like them or hate them, I don't have an alternative to steroids". That lack of choice induces frustrated statements like "I'm not in control".

As if steroids were not a big enough concern, "we elevate other patients to cyclosporin as a desperate means of calming down their inflammation". Cyclosporin is the drug used to prevent organ rejection in transplant patients. It's a "potentially toxic drug and is only used as a last resort". However, there are times when doctors feel "it is necessary". Basically they feel "the patient's immune system has gone wrong and we have to curb its activity". On the positive side, I worked with a young lady who spoke to me half way through her three month programme of cyclosporin. "I finally have relief from the itching that has plagued me all my life. But what do I do when they need to stop the drug? The eczema and itching will just come back, won't they?" In equal parts, she was relieved at the benefits of being on such a powerful immune-suppressing drug and justifiably concerned that the relief could easily be temporary.

Wet-wrapping of children, especially babies, is another tool used to manage severe eczema. The parents of one little girl told me "we wet-wrap her at 7 when we put her to bed and then redo it at 11 when we're ready for bed". They needed to redo the process because "her damaged skin oozes so much under the wrapping". Sadly, they had no choice as "she scratches herself so much in her sleep that she's had repeated blood poisoning".

Another issue young mothers in particular find especially annoying is comments from members of the public on how to "fix" the child's red skin. "I know they mean well" said one mother, "but I didn't ask for their opinion. It's really intrusive and I feel they're criticising my parenting skills". It seems that equally unwelcome are "the people who stare at my child's red skin and then whisper among themselves". That leads some mothers to becoming embarrassed in public and "being embarrassed about your child is a really horrible feeling". When this becomes unbearable, it can lead to a level of social exclusion where the parents are "too scared to go out in case we are judged for our child's bad skin condition".

Great variety is covered in the comments I hear about schools. Occasionally a parent says "the school is really supportive. They've taught the other children that eczema can't be caught from our child. They understand the need for products to be applied throughout the day and go out of their way to ensure it happens".

Sadly, such comments are extremely rare. It's far more common to hear "the school doesn't care. They won't find time to work with our child".

School can be a wonderful place for a child, or a terrible one. Many children with obvious eczema are "shunned by other children". One mother was extremely upset as she detailed "the bullying my child is subjected to by other children. My little girl is really itchy and spends most of her time at school scratching her red skin". Of great relevance was the way this mother felt "the teachers do nothing to reduce the bullying".

Since atopic eczema is said to have a genetic component and "run in families", an element of self-imposed parental guilt can develop. One pair of young parents who knew I had extensive knowledge on eczema were shedding tears when they asked "have we done this to our baby boy?" Both parents were atopic as one had hay fever and the other was asthmatic. They had read of "a 90% likelihood that the baby will have eczema if both parents are atopic". They were really frustrated at being "unable to do anything about it!" They knew the statistic prior to the child's birth and "did everything to prevent the eczema. But we failed. It came anyway as we were told it would". What really seemed to be upsetting them was "being so completely out of control. There is nothing we can do other than let it happen and manage it. We would prefer to end it but we don't know how".

"So many other children grow out of eczema but ours hasn't" is an often heard comment. It seems to put added pressure on parents who "seriously begin to question our parenting skills. Is there something we're missing; perhaps a clue from those children who have ended their eczema?"

One young father who is a researcher in the field of medical immunology, said "I read the technical medical journals and find conflicting views. Some say the skin inflammation is the primary factor and others say the inflammation is the skin's way of reacting to something they haven't determined yet. I just can't find the place to start and all that technical information confuses me even more".

Seeking solace from internet research brings its own type of frustration. Many parents stop researching "as it was just confirming how little control I have over my child's skin problem". The views expressed on blogs, in almost every forum, and on official websites are "so negative". One lady summed it up by saying "I obviously can't do anything to stop the eczema so I just have to manage it as they keep telling me". However, this tenacious woman added "I continue to search the net in the desperate hope that something positive will pop out of the screen". She had been nursing that dream for years.

"Stop scratching" is an instruction many eczema victims say they hate to hear. Ironically, I've had parents say they hate themselves for telling their child to "stop scratching". They know saying that doesn't do any good and is often counterproductive. One mother who was trained in psychology added "The really annoying thing is that I know saying "don't scratch" just induces scratching. Yet I keep saying it even though I know"!

"Being told of the 'atopic march' just deadened our hope". It's a term used to describe the way people with atopic eczema tend to also develop asthma and/or hay fever. "When our child was diagnosed with eczema, rather than help us beat that disease they simply warned us to prepare ourselves for asthma and hay fever. They convinced us it was inevitable so now we're just waiting in dread. That really frustrates us by reinforcing how little control we have. It brings on a presumption of helplessness".

Stress is a word often heard with eczema. Some say "flare-ups are brought on by stress" while others feel "flare-ups cause stress". Some say both. Sadly, they're all correct.

Eczema discussions often centre on products applied to the damaged skin. In many eczema support groups I've taken part in, parents list the products they've tried. None of the products had ended the eczema yet parents who heard of a product they hadn't tried yet, said they were "going to give it a try". A statement often heard in that setting is "I've tried everything and nothing works". Another is "I'm so desperate I'll try anything".

One of the topics discussed tends to be how a "product helped for a while, then seemed to be causing the eczema to get worse, and then seemed to help again". When that is followed by "Has anyone else found that?" you will witness one of the few times there is overwhelming agreement.

"The cost of products can be terrible". Some are prescription products which "lessens the cost for those who have free prescriptions". For everyone else the eczema brings an unwanted financial burden. There are "hidden costs like needing to remove the oily products from clothes and bedding". When the eczema worsens, "as it does for those most affected" there can be an "ever escalating list of products required to manage the disease".

In ironic contrast, I regularly hear that there "are too few products designed for people with eczema". "Given how many millions of us have eczema, you'd think companies would make more products just for us". Those with eczema in the scalp can find "shampoos are too aggressive". Washing up liquid can "make my hand eczema worse".

Many hours each day can be required to "apply the products and manage the disease". It's often said that "eczema rules our family's daily routine".

Several parents have told me they had "to go against my parental instincts" when following the process of managing their child's eczema. This was particularly relevant when the child "screamed when the moisturisers and emollients were applied". Wet-wrapping of children is reserved for the worst cases and one mother said "it was really heart-wrenching when she screamed. It was obvious the products hurt her skin but I was given no choice other than apply them".

A statement I find particularly problematic is "the doctor keeps prescribing products I say make my child scream". Many parents feel the "products seem to fuel the inflammation but we can't get that across to the doctor".

Eczema results in "a really serious loss of sleep" for both affected children and their parents. Tired children "have trouble concentrating at school" and teachers can "sense the negative impact it has on the child's performance". When that leads to exam results below the child's true potential "the consequences of eczema can be devastating and life-long".

Recently I've had a couple say "our dog now has eczema. Can it spread from people to animals?" I let them know dogs can have eczema but it won't spread between humans and animals, just as it won't spread between people.

I think that's enough to show readers how the problems people share about eczema tend to be common experiences. I'm told "it helps to know we're not being singled out by the disease." Nice as that may be, it's very little consolation for the "prolonged misery".

EXeczema® Success

Georgia Smith

Our daughter, Georgia, is 11 and has always had dry, eczema-prone skin that we were managing using a combination of steroid creams and emollients. Her elbows and knees were often extremely sore and her back was incredibly dry and irritated easily.

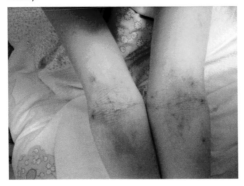

As Georgia went through primary school, so she and her fellow pupils became more conscious of her eczema and she would cover it with her jumper; only to get too hot and rub her skin through the material.

Despite our best efforts, we were fighting a losing battle. No matter how much thick emollient we used, particularly on her back, five minutes later it felt like sandpaper again, often accompanied by long, angry scratch marks across her shoulder blades.

We knew that what we were doing wasn't working. But until we met Harley, we hadn't even considered that we may have been perpetuating the eczema.

Harley gave us the confidence of knowing that Georgia's skin would stay clean and bacteria-free while we weaned her off steroids and emollients. He has also been brilliant at making the process exciting and unintimidating for her – that she's his special 'guinea pig' (music to Georgia's ears - she loves guinea pigs!).

He helped us appreciate how it was all part of her. Rather than seeing the red patches as damaged skin, we came to realise her skin was actually doing what it should be doing to protect her from the products. It took a leap of faith to stop using the products in the hope that her skin would heal itself!

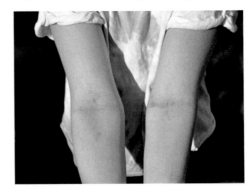

Georgia's back quickly became smooth and eczema-free, as did her legs. Her arms have been more of a challenge, but even there she is 100% better. In our eyes the eczema has gone; it's now just the process of minimising the physical harm done by scratching, which became a habit over the years. She loved Harley's visits when he brought a new 'potion' for her to try. He didn't give up on her scratching habit even though the eczema was long gone. When Georgia gave him this card we couldn't believe how much he treasured it! He even begged Georgia to include it here.

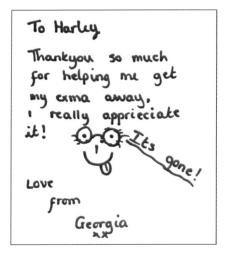

We have always been very skin-aware and done everything we could to avoid her eczema following her into her teen years. With Harley's help, we now have a daughter who can grow up eczema-free.

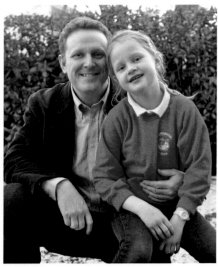

CHAPTER 3

Awaken the issues

What are the practical issues arising from the feelings presented in the previous chapter? What consequences arise from the eczema's existence? What questions arise from the apparent inconsistencies? This chapter provides some of the answers. And it offers a lot more questions.

The visible symptoms of eczema are seen on the skin. However, as those closely associated with eczema know so well, there are many other symptoms *below* the skin. The imbalance is a reflection of the *whole person*. The person's skin affects them and they affect their skin.

Some children have visibly dry skin the day they are born. That's fascinating as they had been immersed in fluid within the womb for months. Within hours of being exposed to air, these children have dry skin. What's going on? Their skin should be saturated with water, soaked, yet it's dry.

Skin is designed to let water from inside the person pass through to the outside. The question for now is whether this dry skin on one-day-old children is caused by too little water passing through the skin, or too much? Either way, one or more of the numerous commercial moisturisers available will probably be applied to the tiny baby's dry skin. These products are intended to produce a water-proof layer to trap the water passing outwards through the skin. The theory says the more these products are applied, the more moisture will be trapped within the skin. Yet the skin of these children remains dry, despite the moisturisers. The children enter a cycle where dry skin and moisturisers become associated. With the moisturisers, the skin remains dry. Without the moisturisers, the skin remains dry. That raises questions, doesn't it? Could it be that the moisturisers are not moisturising? Wouldn't that be interesting for our understanding of how to manage dry skin?

Some of these children with dry skin are diagnosed with eczema; sometimes as early as the first days of life. Why? Is the cause of that eczema coming from inside the skin? If so, it could have been happening *in utero*, while the child was in the womb. Or is the eczema being caused from outside the skin? If so it can only have begun since the child was born.

When eczema is diagnosed in the first days of life, timing becomes very relevant. Did the imbalance actually begin before or after birth? Since we know the holistic 'whole person' approach is warranted, must we face the reality that it could be a bit of both; before *and* after birth? That is certainly the situation for those babies who have eczema diagnosed on day one of their lives. Then we are challenged by the definition of eczema being a chronic condition, even though those who say it's chronic don't specify a minimum time period for their use of the word chronic. Certainly very few would say one day can be chronic. This is the sort of dilemma many people avoid. It raises questions for which they have no simple answers, making it a lot easier to move on without facing the issue presented by these children.

I feel that bypasses a great opportunity. Even though each child went through the stresses of the birth process, it is still the same person that progressed from being a foetus before birth to a baby. Therefore, a one-day old baby can have a chronic skin condition if that had been going on in the womb. Nobody would have seen its skin when it was in the mother, so we can't say whether its skin was reddened before birth. There is, however, no reason why it should not be as the immune system is active before birth.

The advantage of raising this issue lies in exercising our thought processes. When we're considering genuine eczema *in utero* we can discount most of the environmental factors which cause contact dermatitis. They simply won't reach the foetus when it's inside the mother. Obviously the mother makes the fluids which surround the foetus in the uterus so some external factors affecting the mother can affect the foetus via the fluids. For now I would like to take the simplified view of discounting those rare entities.

We have a situation where a foetus surrounded by fluid has a 'dry skin' in contact with those fluids. There won't be any water passing outwards through the skin because the foetus is immersed in liquid. However there can be changes in the skin which become an issue as soon as the baby is in air, immediately after its birth. The skin of all newborn babies goes through rapid changes in the days after birth. When they are born, the pH of the skin is close to neutral reflecting that of the fluid they had been in just hours before. Over several days the skin becomes progressively more acidic until it reaches the normal range of between pH 5 and 6.

The constituents of any liquid used to wash newborn babies is of vital importance. If the detergency is too high it can affect the natural fats in the delicate skin and prevent the baby from forming and maintaining a fully functional skin barrier, the layer within the skin which regulates the rate at which water passes out of the skin. Some chemicals such as sodium lauryl sulphate which are commonly used in skincare products have been proven to be particularly damaging to the skin barrier. That negative effect is even significant on healthy adult skin so you might imagine how damaging such chemicals can be on the skin of day-old babies.

Applying oil to the skin can also be damaging if you use the wrong oil. Olive oil has been proven to significantly damage the skin barrier leading to the suggestion that it should not be used on the skin of children, either as a skin moisturiser or as a massage medium. A peer-reviewed medical article which is about to be published shows that sunflower oil is also detrimental and warrants further study. Mineral oil will penetrate damaged skin decreasing skin barrier effectiveness leading to increased skin dryness.

If the skin barrier is suboptimal, more water will flow out and the skin will feel dry. Dry skin has tiny, usually invisible, cracks in the outer surface. Those cracks will make the babies more susceptible to **Product Maintained Dermatitis**, a new phrase I created and will be describing in subsequent chapters. That will help explain where their eczema came from, what keeps it going and why they have repeated flare-ups. It also provides the clue on how to end the eczema and stop it coming back.

It's said that 20% of children develop eczema during their first year of life. That's one in five, a staggeringly high proportion. To put it in perspective, have you ever seen a horror movie where the producer set out to harm 20% of our babies? I haven't. It's simply too horrendous to contemplate. Yet that's what's happening in our own society; in real life. Something we are doing to those tiny babies has made real life more shocking than the horror movies.

Once children have eczema, their imbalance can take a number of practical paths.

1. In **most** of them, the eczema ends and never comes back. Their skin returns to the correct balance.

2. For **some**, their eczema remains slight with inconvenient itchy areas in the folds of their elbows and knees. This mild eczema can continue for many years before it ends.

3. In a **few**, the eczema becomes severe and requires very active medical intervention which may escalate to wet-wrapping to prevent night-time scratching. In the most extreme cases, cyclosporin may be used to stop the highly intense immune reaction.

I would like you to look at the proportions mentioned in each of those paths. In the first, *most* of the children end their eczema. In the second, *some* have ongoing minor eczema. The key word in the third is *few*. That's a decreasing proportion; *most — some — few*.

Therefore the natural default in children who develop eczema is to end it permanently. That allows me to raise an important question.

What keeps the rest in eczema?

Something is holding children in groups 2 and 3 in the state of imbalance, a very unnatural state. Something is being done to those children to maintain the imbalance. What is it?

In a tiny proportion, they lack the gene for making filaggrin, a protein essential for their skin to work properly. It means they can't make a functional *skin barrier*, the layer in the skin which balances the rate at which water passes out through their skin. For those lacking this gene, it's possible they will always have reddened damaged skin; they may always have eczema. Serious as that is for the unfortunate individuals, they are a tiny minority. The only good bit of news is how they have provided valuable insights into how the skin barrier is created and maintained.

It would be a terrible shame if the sad plight of those lacking this gene came to impede our thinking for the vast majority of eczema sufferers who have perfectly functional versions of that gene. For them, something else is going on.

Skin is our outer barrier to the world and as such is pretty tough. It works well. Yet it's worth knowing that each individual step in making tough skin is a very *delicate* process. All this happens within the skin so it's protected from the outside world. But what if the problem is within the skin itself? That is where a lot of the inflammation of eczema happens; inside the skin.

Inflammation is an incredibly complex process which causes a high number of potentially hazardous chemicals to be made *within* the skin. Those chemicals are there to defend the patient from whatever the inflammation is trying to defeat and remove. But what if that chemical warfare 'battle' is going on just where you had hoped the delicate processes of making vital skin ingredients was happening? It's quite simple. The delicate processes suffer and the production of proteins and fats needed to generate healthy skin can not proceed well. When that happens, the inflamed skin cannot make a fully functional skin barrier. When the eczema is mild, a slightly suboptimal skin barrier is made. When it's severe, the skin barrier is severely impaired.

In relation to the filaggrin protein and it being used to generate a good skin barrier, the effect of chronic inflammation can be the same as a faulty gene not being able to make the protein at all. The resultant eczema is basically the same regardless of how it came about. Inflamed skin with a poor skin barrier will be red, oozing, itchy and result in misery. It's eczema, however it came about.

Rather than delving into the incredible complexities of gene expression and inflammation biomechanics, I want to concentrate on the simple fact that red, oozing, itchy, skin is just that. I want to concentrate on how to end eczema and prevent it coming back. Details of exactly what is happening at the molecular level when the eczema is in full flow can be found in the better medical libraries around the world. Very few people venture there. Believe me, I rarely see more than a few people when I settle into the library for one of my research days. The value in this book derives from trusting me to 'liberate' the most useful gems of wisdom and present them in a usable form.

I would now like to expand our focus to all ages with eczema, from the extremely young to the elderly. Skin alters with age yet eczema affects people of all ages despite those age-related variations in skin. The latter provide clues for those of us seeking to consider skin and eczema at the molecular levels. For those people who are content to leave such cerebral exercises to the likes of me, eczema can be viewed as basically the same condition regardless of the victim's age.

The same applies to ethnic origin. There are very obvious differences in the skin between ethnic groups. However, my contribution to the eczema debate shows those differences are not relevant to how we end eczema. The differences actually helped me discover the secret which allowed people in all the major ethnic groups to end their eczema and prevent it coming back.

Each individual eczema sufferer has their baseline level of eczema. On top of that they have flare-ups. It's also likely they have joyful periods of freedom from eczema. Those happy times are followed by relapses. That's the eczema cycle and they're repeatedly told it can't be cured.

Yet it's well known that most children with eczema grow out of it. All those children *end* their eczema. I will repeat what I consider to be a key question.

What keeps the rest in eczema?

Sometimes their flare-ups can be traced to certain events. For one young boy, his flare-ups happened after his school swimming sessions. Initially it seemed to be related to the fact that his school had chosen to prevent the children having a shower after they left the pool. Ironically there were no flare-ups when he went swimming in the same pool with his family, even when he didn't shower after his swim. So the problem was not the chlorine in the pool water or whether he showered or not after the swim. The details of what was happening to him, which will be revealed later, helped generate the novel and positive thoughts in this book.

Stress is a major inducement to flare-ups. Since stress is such a subjective matter, it has proven useful to examine deeply the psychology of how stress and eczema inter-relate. That subject could form the basis of a complete book so here I will only discuss some of the factors which confirm the relationship between stress and eczema flare-ups.

A major contributor to the stress is frustration at the statement that eczema can't be cured. Some prefer to call this reality. Regardless of how you want to see it, repeatedly hearing that eczema can't be cured weighs heavily. Repeatedly telling patients that eczema can't be cured weighs heavily on some doctors. Being told that all you can do is manage it simply adds to the burden and stress. In effect, you're being told there's no sense in even trying to do better. There's no hope.

That's why I prefer to classify such advice as pervading negativity. In saying that, I am deliberately offering an alternative view to those of the national eczema support groups and the medical profession. As with any state of mind, if you believe the critical word is **can't** you will be right. While people remain in that state of mind, they can't end eczema. And they don't. The only option remaining to them is to manage it. That decreases the likelihood that they will seek clues even when those clues are readily available. After all, why bother looking for clues if you believe they can't exist? Why stress yourself by hoping for something better? Why dream of taking control?

If the preceding paragraph infuriates you, I apologise unreservedly for upsetting you and suggest you leave this book for another time. My chosen purpose in life is to bring health and happiness. Everything I do is directed to that purpose, including writing this book. It is a reality that not everyone is ready to encompass the health and happiness I value. Or perhaps it's more a case of them not being ready *yet*. This book will be useful to most readers now. For others, it will be useful at some time in the future.

I value choice and like to help people see the choices available to them. The pervading negativity about eczema suggests you have no choice. All you can do is manage it. Only being given one option offers no choice.

I add the option that you can end it. End the eczema. Why would I, with all my qualifications, including in psychology, offer something so different from that offered by the recognised authorities? Please allow me to answer that with a question.

If you are seeking a positive outcome, do you feel it's most likely to be found with those who say "we can't" or those who say "we did"?

Those who say "we can't" are working with those who remain in eczema. Those who say "we did" are the ones who ended their eczema. And they did it despite hearing the statement "we can't".

Fortunately, the vast majority of eczema sufferers end their eczema and only a minority remain in the state of skin imbalance. Many of those who ended their eczema are delighted to share details on how they achieved it. All their positivity is available to those who seek it. That is where I sought details which allowed me to develop my clues.

I found that quite easy as I'd had bad eczema when I was a young man. As my clinical skills developed and my technical knowledge grew, I found a way of ending my eczema. My skin remains sensitive so now I have decades of experience in how to prevent eczema in sensitive skin. That helped me form the appropriate questions and those questions revealed very useful answers.

I firmly believe the answers are out there. All I need do is find the questions.

In contrast, those who don't believe the answers are out there will have little incentive to seek the questions. Or perhaps there is a disinclination to value the questions others are asking. The answers are then not available, even though they are there delivering positive outcomes for others.

This vital distinction rests on a choice of words. "We can't" and "we did" represent different outcomes, don't they?

It's therefore appropriate to examine another word that's prominent in the eczema dialogue. Manage. When you manage eczema you're acknowledging that it will keep going. Would the outcome change if the word *manage* was replaced with *maintain*?

Interesting, isn't it? Spend a little time thinking back on the advice you have received about eczema. Perhaps you are one of those who gives advice on eczema. Would the disease outcome be the same if the word "manage" was replaced with "maintain"?

Might *manage* mean *maintain*?

If so, the way people feel trapped within eczema becomes justified. The isolation they feel is warranted. They know of many other people who've ended their eczema and moved on, yet they find themselves left isolated in a bad state of confusion.

Are you being advised to maintain the eczema? Perhaps there is an even more disturbing question. Could you be *advising* people to maintain eczema?

The basic choice I present in this book is to:

1. carry on the same way and manage eczema or

2. make small, easy changes, and end eczema.

You may be very experienced at the first. The great news is that most people who've proven they can manage eczema readily progress to achieve the second choice — when they learn how. Many favourable experiences from the second group are shared here.

EXeczema® Success

Susan Ellis – the 'cool, clean, cover and carry on' strategist.

Having suffered with painful, debilitating and persistent hand eczema for over 25 years, I thought I would never be free from this horrible condition. Visits to my family doctor always resulted in multiple prescriptions for various emollients and steroids, none of which seemed effective and, indeed, often seemed to exacerbate things.

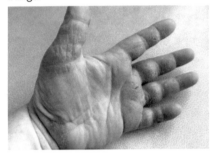 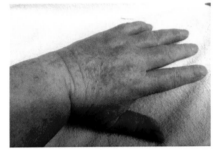

I make delicate silver jewellery and sell it in the local craft market of our university city. People from all over the world like the jewellery and I always wondered what effect my horrible looking hands were having. Dr Harley had known me for years and his wife Dr Anne-Marie had bought my jewellery. When I mentioned my hands during one of their visits to my stand, they asked if it would help to have healthy skin. In hindsight, I appreciate how they never attempted to push their knowledge on me. It was available if I wanted it.

I was told that by following the EXeczema principals, my condition could be resolved in three months. I was sceptical but having tried everything else without success and feeling depressed and despondent, I was willing to try. Harley found a way to make a little fun by us setting a date of Christmas 'for the impossible'. That would represent the busiest time of my year when I would be making the most jewellery. It would be the time when my hands suffered the greatest chemical insult.

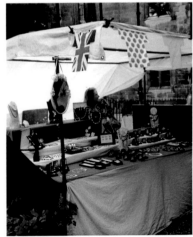

So I accepted. The theory made sense - the very creams and steroids prescribed to help my condition were maintaining the eczema and perpetuating the cycle of broken, inflamed skin.

And so, I put away all the creams and started using Dr Harley's products. I learned that chronic eczema was not just a physical condition but also a state of mind. I realised just how much I was preoccupied with rubbing, scratching, picking and scrutinising my hands. I would like to say the process of change was easy, but it was not. One thing I had in my favour was the way Harley and Anne-Marie visited my stand every Saturday to see how I was progressing and offer support. They knew that as an ex-nurse I understood biology. It was soon apparent they expected me to find the answers I needed. To be more exact, they were guiding me to finding the questions most relevant to me. I now know they were gently coaching me to realise I was in control - something I had never considered for a quarter of a century.

The thing I found most difficult to contend with was the dryness that developed as my skin healed. The first two months were a roller coaster of progress and relapse. But I didn't give up. I found that if I had an itch I could soothe it with immersing my hands in cold water. If I had little broken areas, simply covering with a sticking plaster or simple dressing took away the itch and stopped further trauma. I dealt with the dryness by wearing latex-free gloves which helped retain the moisture naturally being lost through my broken skin. I washed my hands frequently with the Foam Wash and rinsed them, at least every couple of hours, and then immediately put on a fresh pair of gloves.

Repeating this regime and by using only the Dr Harley's Foam Wash throughout the day, meant that my skin had the chance to repair itself and more importantly, without the itch, dryness and sores, I could get on with my day and barely gave my skin a second thought. After just one week of finding this regime, my skin was transformed. I have healthy new skin on my hands and the difference this has made to my life is enormous.

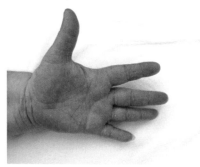 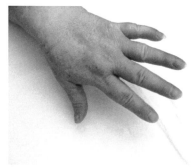

I continue to maintain healthy skin by completely avoiding contact with chemicals, soaps and detergents (keeping a pair of gloves to hand is useful). I use only NewGenn Foam Wash and always carry a little bottle whenever I go out or on holiday. If I do get an occasional itch, I just act fast, and put into action the 'cool, clean, cover and carry on' strategy.

My skin no longer controls me. I now know that I am in control.

CHAPTER 4

Look to action

Could *managing* eczema be *maintaining* eczema?

Those who've ended their eczema all took action. They succeeded. Others didn't and they remained with eczema.

I gain delight from those who succeed but my knowledge grows regardless of the patient outcome. It's just as important to know why someone chose to remain with eczema as it is to learn from those who chose to take action and achieve healthy skin.

Given that my chosen purpose in life is to bring health and happiness, I like to avoid pushing anyone in any direction. I prefer to attract them to take action which is likely to bring them health and happiness. I've found those who are not ready for action, for whatever reasons, gain a lot from watching the people they see taking action. Many of those who are waiting and watching subsequently take action when they've gained enough confidence from seeing the increasing number of positive outcomes achieved by those they're watching.

The best thing we can do for those who choose to watch is give them something exciting to watch.

Let's revisit that question. Does *manage* mean *maintain*?

You will appreciate I present it as a question rather than a statement of fact. The history of medicine is littered with examples of good and logical ideas that proved to be inappropriate. I like readers to appreciate I am fully aware of that fact.

Yet the history of life, including medicine, reveals many instances where substantial progress is made when complexity is replaced by simplicity. As we hear so often, "The simple ones are the best".

If changing ***one letter*** can change patient outcomes, that's simplicity at its best. Would you agree? All will be revealed in the clue chapters.

Eczema is an incredibly complicated condition and a few people may never be able to escape their eczema. Those lacking a specific gene to make vital proteins can't make a complete skin barrier. They may have to live with their eczema as best they can (although I don't believe it's all negative). Some people with severe chronic skin itching for which nobody can find a valid explanation may unfortunately be in the same situation. For now.

Yet the vast majority of people with eczema do not have those underlying problems as their primary issue. Their damaged eczema skin will have trouble making the correct levels of filaggrin protein so their skin barrier effectiveness is less than optimal. Their skin will also be very itchy. But for this group comprising so many millions of eczema sufferers, their primary initiating problem is not centred on such issues. For them, insufficient filaggrin protein and chronic intense itching are the **result** of their eczema. Their eczema is maintained by something else.

In the medical and technical literature there are excellent scientific articles detailing many other cause-and-effect scenarios which result *once eczema is established*. A lot of the evidence centres on what the immune system is doing *during eczema*. Those articles have great value for people like me who seek to understand all we can about the imbalance. They tend to have very little relevance for those who simply seek to end eczema. Delving deep into the confusing complications brings confusing complications. Few surprises there! Simplicity comes from having a single objective.

Most of the people who've shared the positive experiences mentioned here had a single objective; to end eczema.

I chose to offer them the additional prize of knowing how to prevent eczema coming back. To achieve that, they needed to gain a small amount of new knowledge to develop a useful practical understanding of eczema. They had to decide they wanted that new knowledge.

I was guiding them on a journey from a bad place called eczema to a good place I call EXeczema, the time *after* eczema.

The really important point is how they *wanted* to come on the journey. That sounds simple and it is. First, I needed to arouse their interest in somewhere different, somewhere they felt was better. It was vital to have them decide that where they were was somewhere they preferred to leave; to instil confidence that a better place existed and reaching it was well within their capacity.

I choose to use the simple analogy of a path.

They know many others have benefitted from following the path and the task is to have them appreciate how they can do the same. Such a process requires them to take many small steps, each fuelled by confidence they progressively develop when each tiny action step provides positive reward.

There is one special secret; a choice they really come to value. Whenever they want, they can step to the side of the path and pause their journey. For many people this decision to step aside for a while is the most important action they take in the whole journey. Take a look at the picture on the front cover — there are seats beside the path for those who wish to spend time sitting and watching. That is important in this path analogy. When they are ready, they WANT to step onto the path again and progress at their own speed to their desired outcome.

Every person is different. Everyone with eczema is different. I am simply showing them a common path, the one taken by those who have ended their eczema. Some individuals sprint along that path at breathtaking speed and reach their goal of healthy skin in less than two weeks. I tend to be dazzled by them! Delighted, but dazzled, as I'm not a sprinter. Others take their time, some even opting to take months. There is no judgement in the timeframe they choose. I like to offer them control over their rate of progress. If that happens to be a zero rate and they opt to remain with eczema, listening to them has value in the overall scheme of ending eczema.

I've chosen to take my EXeczema campaign global to show many millions of people this path. Imagine the turmoil if all those many millions decided to walk that path tomorrow. They wouldn't fit! So I actually WANT people to choose their own rate, including the moment they begin. I rely on many people NOT beginning the journey as soon as they hear of it. They will come along at their own pace when they're ready. Or they won't. They are in control now.

I like to find time to spend with individuals who haven't started yet. They have a lot to teach someone like me who listens. Others prefer to begin the journey and seek support when they 'step off the path' for a while. The beauty of the path analogy is that both of these groups gain the confidence they seek by watching others who are progressing along the path.

There are always a tiny number of individuals who chose to go backwards on the path; go back to the starting point and deliberately remain with eczema. That is the correct action for them; they are doing the best they can with the resources they have available. Judgement is left for others.

Regardless of where a person is on the path they have something to offer everyone else. We have ample numbers at the end of the path and many of those have actively shared their experiences. Around the world there are many millions who have yet to hear of the path. Imagine the wealth of knowledge they collectively hold from their experiences of life. It would be wonderful to have them all share, wouldn't it? All we need do is listen.

I like to repeat that it's just as important to hear why someone won't start the journey as it is to know why someone completed the journey.

The purpose of this book is to let people know what choices are available. In the simplest terms, they can maintain eczema or end it. Each of those choices needs to be expanded, taking care to remain within the realms of simplicity.

The choice to take no action and remain with eczema is one many people select. This is perfectly understandable in the context of what they've been told repeatedly, sometimes over many years and even decades. When authorities you trust repeatedly say "eczema can't be cured" you can come to believe it. When people are content and happy with the constraints placed upon them by that belief, all I tend to offer is the addition of two words; "by us".

Then you have "eczema can't be cured *by us*". As you can imagine, the authorities I'm referring to are extremely unlikely to add those two words. So why do I choose to? Because it helps people see that the constraints are created and imposed by the authorities; they are NOT constraints eczema sufferers have created for themselves. The person can still opt to choose to be personally constrained by the authority's constraints. When they do, I leave them to appreciate the subtle difference my two added words deliver. The authorities are correct to say *they* can't cure eczema. That is a very long way from saying the individual sufferer can't.

Once the relevance of those two words is fully appreciated, a new perspective to seek options and choices becomes available. That opens new opportunities and most take action to grasp those opportunities they had not been offered before. Some don't and that is the correct decision for them at the time.

One choice is to set out with intent to end eczema. That requires certain specific actions. Fortunately the whole journey is a sequence of small actions so the person is never at undue risk. They are fully aware that the greatest risk to their health and happiness is to stay with eczema and remain in the state of imbalance constrained by mental boundaries set by someone else.

I've gone to great lengths to ensure none of those who want to take action ever have to take a big action. The intention is to make the transition from eczema to EXeczema very gentle. The outcome is dramatic, even though it comes about through many undramatic steps.

If you are one of the many who've decided to take action to end eczema, I welcome you onto the path to EXeczema success.

EXeczema® Success

Max takes the fast route – once his parents had the clues!

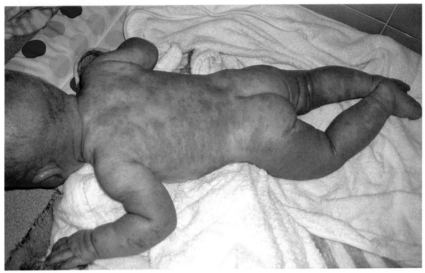

As a tiny baby Max had terrible eczema. We followed all the medical advice and applied the skin products as directed. It was incredibly hard to just watch our baby boy go red. We hated what we saw but medical advice is there to be followed.

In due course Max progressed to the full set of atopic diseases with asthma and hay fever, plus becoming hyper-allergic to certain foods. He always was and is still a really happy little boy but as parents we were at a loss.

Over the years we learned more and by the time Max was three we had the eczema under control. We could manage it so Max only had the typical areas of itchy redness in his elbows and on the back of his knees. We were still following the advice to apply moisturisers, emollients and various strengths of hydrocortisone cream depending on the severity of his rashes. Unfortunately, it seemed the more we applied the more Max scratched. But compared to when he was red all over we were content with being able to manage it.

As a baby Max had bad reflux and struggled to feed, so was put on a hypoallergenic milk formula called Neocate, which really helped, but we were told we should expect Max to always have eczema. Then something really simple happened and within two weeks Max had clear skin with no eczema. You can see the difference in the photos below.

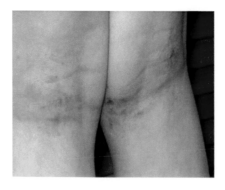
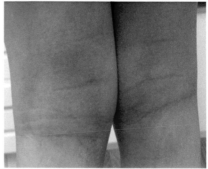

As you can guess, we met Dr Harley. He explained his ideas and with our intense experience of childhood eczema it was a huge relief to have the eczema explained for the first time. He easily builds good bonds with children and Max liked him immediately, which made it much easier for us to introduce a new skincare regime. The fact that Harley's products came out as bubbles made bath time fun, especially when we told Max that Harley had a bubble factory! Prior to this we avoided bubble bath as so many of the bath products aimed at children seemed to make his skin worse.

In the years since we ended the eczema, Max rarely has skin rashes and any outbreaks are very minor and are usually as a result of charging round the garden and being a normal little boy! Every rash was washed with the foam washes and none turned into eczema. The knowledge we gained from Harley and the suggestions he gave us, were very easy to use to Max's benefit — and our relief.

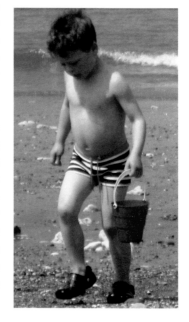

Max remains very allergic to certain foods, in particular, fish and peanuts. He continues to suffer from hay fever but is currently being treated with Stalerol; fingers crossed it has the same effect as 'Harley's bubbles'. However he does not have eczema, despite all the warnings we were given. He is undoubtedly atopic and may always remain so but he no longer has eczema. We believe this proves Harley's statement that the Atopic March does not have to be permanent as the eczema can be ended by utilising his three simple clues.

Meeting Harley was a chance event when he welcomed us as new arrivals into the village. It's the sort of thing he does. Being the person he is, Harley did not tell us of his work and it was another chance event which led us to hearing his ideas on eczema. With nothing to loose, we decided to try Harley's regime and didn't use any other products during this time. Initially Max's skin seemed to get better and then around day 9 it got worse and as bits started to scab over and Max scratched, it really tested our resolve, but we stuck with it. Amazingly after 13 days Max had no eczema! You can imagine our relief. We don't see Harley all that often now but every time we do Max's face lights up. We look forward to our lives without eczema and a new lifelong friendship.

Sharing Max's EXeczema success will hopefully help other families end the misery.

Jill and Tim Wildish, Cambridgeshire, England.

CHAPTER 5

Encouragement

What would your ideal solution to eczema be like? Can you imagine life without eczema; all that misery gone, all that time saved, all that new health and happiness?

With that end target in mind, can you describe what you would want in order to reach it? The secret to the EXeczema programme reveals itself when people WANT to take the next small step. They are drawn forward by their vision of life after eczema.

You will generate your own incentives for each successive small step. How do you achieve that? What allows you to create all those tiny incentives whenever you want them? After all, not so long ago, hadn't you heard there was no point in even trying to escape eczema?

Many changes happen as someone begins the EXeczema journey. For many it's a growing realisation that they are replacing their fear of eczema with confidence. The confidence builds control. Knowing they finally understand the imbalance, what was keeping it going and what allowed it to come back each time, puts them in control. Usually for the first time.

This change happens with all those who succeed, including doctors who advise sufferers. You realise eczema is a sequence of logical events, a sequence that can be broken. You recognise that the word *atopic,* as in atopic eczema, equates to a lack of understanding. It's used in that context because nobody could understand why the immune system created all that inflammation which was acting against the patient.

You come to realise the inflammation is not acting against the patient at all; it's acting against something being put in contact with the patient. It's doing what needs to be done to defend the patient against something foreign, something non-human.

Would it help to understand the difference, to know why the word atopic represents defeatism?

Think back to the many times when you heard the word atopic being used in relation to eczema. If you are a doctor, consider the situations in which you relied on that word atopic. Was it when you were trying to help a patient with persistent eczema? Could it have been patients who often had phases with no eczema and then saw it come back with a vengeance? You were fully justified in not understanding what was going on, weren't you? Would it help if you gained a little new knowledge that allows a completely new perspective, one which provides a full understanding of eczema? One that put you in control of eczema allowing you to end it? Take a little time to consider how that would change your life as a doctor.

Be generous; you owe it to yourself. Find some time to do just that. What would it be like?

Parents, if your child suffers from eczema, consider a similar outcome. Take a few moments to realise how your family's life will change when you understand eczema to the point where you end it. Imagine the health and happiness stemming from your new control.

If you are an older eczema sufferer in charge of your own balance, take a deep breath, clear your mind of all that old negative misery and refresh it with pleasant thoughts of healthy skin.

The little bit of knowledge you want is coming after this chapter. To gain the most from that knowledge, it's best to reinforce the point you have reached. Perhaps without even appreciating it, in reading to this point you have progressed beyond needing to accept words like atopic. You are now ready to know what it is that eluded you before.

Now another profound little question. If it's so simple, why was it missed by so many people?

Cast your mind back to how often you heard the statement "eczema can't be cured"? If you're a doctor or someone involved in managing eczema, how often did you say it? When you hear it often enough, or say it often enough, it becomes your reality. Add to that your experience of how long the eczema persisted and if it ever went away, how it came back. That is personal reality and it reinforced the view that eczema can't be cured. For you, in those situations, it wasn't cured. Your reality is fully justified.

Do you see how one word helped generate limiting beliefs? Can't is a powerful word. If you can't you can't! Those saying or hearing "you can't" are doing the best they can with the resources they have available. Remember, I leave judgement for others so there is no judgement here. But there are questions. And consequences.

Parental instincts don't give way to such defeatism without reason. Doctors don't constrain their patients with limiting beliefs without some justification.

Something profound has been happening; something big enough to trap tens of millions of people into a single skin change, all around the world. It induces limiting beliefs of such magnitude that all those millions of people, both sufferers and health providers alike, choose to be controlled by the constraints. They opt to give up their control. There will have been a good reason, won't there?

This is the appropriate moment for you to play a mind game. First, accept the reality of all those people constrained by the limiting belief that you can't cure eczema. They are real and their shared belief is real.

While you are appreciating how real it all is, lift your mind up to sufficient height where you can see all those millions of people with eczema. Relax into it, it's just a mind game. You might want to leave your body down there in the crowd if that represents your reality best. If it suits you better, envisage yourself in your body as having left the group and drifted up to the point of being able to see the others still left with the eczema. The important key is that you achieve the new perspective of being above and separated from the eczema.

Good; that's the best way to do it.

What would it feel like to help those down there, people still constrained by the limiting belief? Remember, in your mind you have separated yourself from their situation; you have a new perspective. It's a mind exercise, yet can you begin to feel what it would be like to actually do it? To actually separate yourself from eczema, prevent it coming back and then help others? Really anchor that good feeling within you. Let it go deep.

While you are up there, take a look to the side and see another group of people. A MUCH LARGER group of people and appreciate they are the ones who've already ended their eczema. All around the world most of those who develop eczema end it, so this groups is huge. You know that group exists. You know they are real. Most of them are willing to help, many have taken action in sharing their experiences here so you can gain from their success. It's a happy group where the limiting belief that you can't cure eczema has been dispelled. There are no constraining boundaries restricting that group.

Now look from one group to the other and back again. Both groups are real; you know that. But one is much smaller. The smaller group has chosen to be constrained by boundaries induced by the limiting belief that eczema can't be cured. The much larger group has taken action to break through the boundaries and live in a happier state without eczema. Safety in numbers is something ingrained into the human psyche and whether you opt to reside in the smaller group, or join the much larger group, is a choice that is now available to you.

Good. Now bring your mind back down to physical reality. If that returns you to the smaller group, the one with boundaries supported by the limiting belief, you have a pleasant surprise. You have positioned yourself at the boundary and gained the choice to break through.

Not yet, but very soon, you will have the knowledge to break through your boundary. You will gain confidence and an appreciation of why many more people have broken through that boundary than are constrained by it. You will soon be a able to achieve greater safety by moving to a group with larger numbers.

You are now making excellent use of my path analogy. During that simple yet profound mind game, you took time away from the misery of eczema. You stepped aside from the path to gain a new perspective. Remember how I mentioned that for some people, the action of stepping aside was the most important action they took on the journey to EXeczema? Now appreciate how easy it was. You simply lifted your mind up, looked to the side to see the other choice and then came back down knowing your new choice was credible.

Some people shy away from such mind games. They say it can't be that simple. They suggest it's damaged skin they're concerned with so why am I emphasising the mind? If those thoughts are trying to influence you, ask yourself a question. Does the limiting belief that eczema can't be cured reside in the skin or the mind? It's the mind, isn't it? You will soon appreciate how the damaged skin of an eczema sufferer is doing a magnificent job of defending the sufferer. The skin is fine and it will heal itself when you allow that to happen.

Eczematous skin is not in some form of self-destruct mode. For many years the vast majority of people who ever had eczema ended it and progressed to normal healthy skin. That was the default situation long before the EXeczema word was introduced.

Their skin was never the controlling factor. It was the limiting belief in their mind which led the skin to need all that inflammation. The skin was performing as it should when it was challenged by some physical onslaught. It was the mind which believed it should keep that onslaught coming. It was the mind which led them to believe all they could do was manage eczema by applying all those products.

Conscious actions come from the mind. Organs like the skin simply react to whatever action the mind has decided to take.

Why do I continue to mention this difference? Because it allows a different perspective. Do you have to tolerate this new way of looking at things? No. You can step aside from the path and stay there. You can reverse your journey and go back to the start and remain with eczema. Remember, you are now in control.

If you're a doctor you can ignore this new way of thinking about eczema and continue to *manage* eczema in your patients. That's what you were expected to do before you read to this point. In many respects that's the easier choice. After all, you see all those patients with persistent eczema come into your clinic. They are your focus. You don't see the much greater number who have ended their eczema and no longer take up your time. So you can easily justify serving those who continue to seek your advice on how to manage their persistent skin changes. Or you could help all those sufferers end their eczema. Not yet, but soon, you will know how. For now, take a moment to ask if the mind game of lifting yourself high above the eczema group gave you a perspective of the other group? You chose a medical career which allows you to help people end their ailments. Eczema is just one of the many imbalances you influence with your advice. Would it be good to have fewer eczema patients and be able to devote all that time to patients with other complaints?

Skin is the organ which leads to most consultations with family doctors and eczema is a high proportion of the skin conditions you see. Imagine how much time you will gain when you end eczema in your patients. There are still many eczema sufferers so you will still have people with eczema seek your advice. Imagine being able to say "Great. It's eczema. I know how to end that".

If you are the parent of a child sufferer, how will you feel when you've used the new knowledge and your child's eczema ends? What comments are you going to get from your friends and family? What would you be able to offer other parents who asked how you did it? How good will that feel?

Now for a really powerful mind game. Since you are reading this, you're likely to be tall enough for young children to look up to you, literally. You are taller than them. Ask yourself how you will feel when those cute little eyes are looking up at you saying "Thank you. My eczema is gone".

Take your time. It's your reward for taking the action and learning how to end eczema. I've had that fantastic experience many times. You've seen real examples between the chapters as you progressed through this book. It really is as wonderful as you imagine it could be. It's something I love to share. Would you like to share it too?

EXeczema® Success

Beeka's own Story by Rebecca Hindle. (Beeka)

When I got rid of my eczema I could finally go out in shorts again, it was just wonderful because when I had eczema I was worried that people would laugh at me so I didn't like to wear shorts and short sleeve tops.

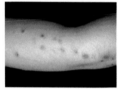

My eczema used to get really horrible over the summer, which made it hard for me on hot nights, additionally if I had a sleepover on that hot night I got really worried my friends would see my arms and legs and laugh at me.

I had to try all kinds of things to cure my eczema such as creams; oils; gloves; bandages and wipes but I had lots of doctors and nurses informing me that light treatment was the way forward. That scared me.

Every night I put the cream on and awoke hoping that it had gone; it hadn't. It was the same every summer. But a long while later I was given a special body wash that helped me tremendously.

I am so glad that my eczema has gone and I can have long nails and not have to worry about people laughing at me and now the things I enjoy are more enjoyable.

No Shadows Behind the Eyes, by Beeka's mother, Karen Hindle

Life would be awful if we had not found NewGenn. We were facing intensive, potentially cancerous light treatment to fix Beeka's skin.

Very scary.

Beeka, 12, dreaded the summer when her eczema would flare up. She hated it when she put shorts on. She'd smile but you could always see the shadows behind her eyes.

Not any more. We had to stop using all the treatments we had been using and effectively do nothing for 14 days. We were given a specific skin wash and wipes to use and that was it. We watched amazed as the angry spots settled down. Now, you know what? We don't do anything at all. We just remain vigilant and bring out the skin wash and wipes if we need to.

For the first time Beeka has long fingernails and enjoys putting on nail varnish.

As I write this she is outside with her brother; they have found a newt in the pond and she calls up to us to go and look. She is sporting a huge smile.

There are no more shadows.

CHAPTER 6

The 3 clues

Now for the three little clues that will help you end eczema. Relax; it's really simple. So simple that most people missed it while they were searching for complications. Over the decades, many millions of people ended eczema without having a PhD, without degrees in complicated methods of disease control.

They just did it.

You'll see the clues they've chosen to share and you'll learn how to do it yourself. The fun begins.

The clues are:

1. Whether a product is ON the skin or IN the skin makes a huge difference.
2. Eczema is a SECOND-level condition.
3. The skin replaces itself every month.

That's it! I will expand on all three so you come to realise why they form the answers to eczema. For now, take a moment to appreciate you will be in control of eczema once you know those three simple clues and begin using them all.

Whether a product is ON the skin or IN the skin makes a huge difference

The best analogy here is to consider a splinter of wood. If it rests ON the skin it has no relevance to the immune system. It's just a piece of foreign material sitting on the skin surface where the immune system does not detect it.

In contrast, consider what happens when that splinter of wood goes IN the skin. It's detected by the immune system because the splinter of wood is foreign to the human body. Inflammation develops around the splinter. Why? Because the immune system is using the inflammation as a tool to expel the splinter.

Since it's working against the splinter, the inflammation is a good thing, isn't it? It's the means by which the immune system is protecting the person from foreign material which should not be where it is.

Simple? Absolutely.

Could you imagine anyone wanting to stop the inflammation which is acting to expel that piece of foreign material? No? I agree, as that would be acting against the interests of the patient. If the skin is left alone to heal itself, the inflammation will expel the splinter and the skin will return to normal. That healthy state is the one which protects the patient best.

Now consider the products applied to skin damaged with eczema. Do those products contain ingredients which are foreign to the human body? Yes. Have a look at the ingredient lists. Apart from aqua (water) the ingredients are all foreign. Individual ingredients may have 'green' credentials but they, and the products in which they are included, are still foreign to the human body.

When such ingredients are placed ON the skin, the immune system does not detect them. There will be no inflammation.

In contrast, consider what happens when such a product goes IN the skin. It's detected by the immune system because the product is foreign to the human body. The result is red inflammation around the product. Why? Because the immune system is using the inflammation as a tool to expel the product.

Does that last paragraph sound familiar? It's virtually the same as the one describing what happens with a splinter IN the skin, isn't it?

Yes, because the immune system will use inflammation to remove anything foreign which it detects IN the skin. Therefore the inflammation is a good thing as it's the person's defence against foreign chemicals being in the skin.

Could you imagine anyone wanting to stop the inflammation which is acting to expel that foreign material? No? I agree, as that would be acting against the interests of the patient. If the skin is left alone to heal itself, the inflammation will expel the product and the skin will return to normal. That healthy state is the one which protects the patient best.

Do you notice more similarities with the foreign splinter example? Keep this in mind as it will help bring the second piece of knowledge into perspective.

How can such products get IN the skin? Weren't they put *ON* the skin? The splinter was easy to understand because it was pushed into the skin. The products were placed gently on the skin. That's perfectly true, so what small piece of information may be missing? The answer is part of the new knowledge.

The skin can have surface cracks which allow products placed ON the skin to go IN the skin. If they go deep enough for the immune system to detect them it will react with inflammation. You would want the immune system to do precisely that, wouldn't you? Yes, because that's how the immune system protects the person from something that should not be there.

That makes it important to know more about skin cracks. Most of them are too small to be seen; they are invisible. However, it has recently been proven that tiny cracks appear *before* the skin feels dry. The technical name for dry skin is xerosis and a feature of xerosis is skin cracks.

Therefore any product put onto dry skin is being placed on skin with cracks. Most of the product will remain ON the skin. Some will go down the cracks becoming IN the skin. If it goes deep enough, you know the immune system will react with red inflammation as it should do. And we should be happy that it does.

Now ask yourself whether any products which are foreign to the human body are ever placed on fine looking skin which feels dry? Yes. Moisturisers. And there's great encouragement from the manufacturers to use the moisturisers as soon as we feel the sensation of dry skin, isn't there?

That was on healthy looking skin which had simply become dry. What about skin that is obviously damaged and red? The cracks may still be invisible yet they are definitely there.

Now consider a red patch of skin which has earned the diagnosis of eczema. You know that is definitely damaged skin. There will be cracks within those red, inflamed, itchy, patches of skin. Can you think of any products which people with eczema are told to put onto those areas of damaged skin? Yes. Emollients.

What would you want the immune system to do when it detects

these foreign materials IN the skin? Would you want it to use inflammation to expel the foreign chemicals? If so, would you want anyone to actively decrease the inflammation that was defending the person? If not, you may value my thoughts in the final chapter where I challenge some treatment paradigms.

Keep in mind that the inflammation in eczema is decreased by drugs like steroids. They are often applied as *steroid creams*. If the inflammation is a good thing defending the patient, using steroids to decrease that defence could be against the patient's best interests. Correct?

However, there are two more vital points. First, steroids tend to be prescribed by doctors and tolerated by eczema sufferers because the steroids reduce the inflammation in eczema. However there is medical evidence that the steroids reduce the ability of new skin cells to make components of the all important skin barrier. When the skin barrier is suboptimal foreign chemicals put ON the skin have a greater chance of going IN the skin. Topical steroids help in one respect and *cause* the problem in another. Interesting, isn't it? A bit frightening too when you realise that vital piece of medical research was published in a top Dermatology journal years ago by very credible people. There is simply no avoiding the facts revealed by this evidence.

For the second point, I would like to suggest that of those two words, *steroid* and *cream*, the latter warrants a lot more concern than it normally receives. The *cream* is viewed by most people as just an inert carrier for the drug. Yet isn't that cream foreign to the human body? When it's applied to patches of damaged skin with cracks, won't some of it go IN the skin provoking the immune system to react against it with inflammation? Yes. So the body is doing a good job in attempting to protect the person from a foreign material which has inadvertently gone IN the skin. The cream can be causing the very inflammation the steroid is intended to stop.

When you are shown how to *manage* eczema, are you told to apply products which could go IN the skin where they will *maintain* the inflammation? In that case, would *manage* equal *maintain*? Are you beginning to imagine a cycle where products cause the disease those same products are used to manage?

Product Maintained Dermatitis is the name I gave to that cycle. It will become even more relevant in a short while.

For now, are you happy that whether a product is ON the skin or IN the skin makes a huge difference? If not, please go back and read this chapter again as the understanding of this fundamental clue is essential before proceeding.

If you are happy to accept the logic within this concept, you have come to your own realisation on the first of the three clues. You're well on your way to understanding eczema, quite possibly for the first time.

You now know why changing one letter is pivotal to understanding eczema. Change the O in On to an I and you have IN. Change one letter and you change the disease outcome. Simple, isn't it?

EXeczema® Success

Barnaby and then Phili

Ever since Barnaby was newborn he often developed a red, blotchy rash that felt very rough all across his tummy. Initially I treated it with an emollient cream from the USA and I thought this was brilliant until I realised that if I didn't put the cream

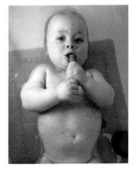

on the rash just came back. It then dawned on me that Barnaby was suffering from Eczema. I was insistent that I didn't want him to be on steroid creams before his first birthday and in conversations with family and friends I discovered Dr Harley Farmer.

I started the EXeczema programme, (much to Barnaby's nursery's disbelief) I persevered (and made them too!) and the result is now a little chap with no eczema and baby soft skin!

Any sight of any redness or roughness I use Dr Harley's fantastic Foam Emollient and in a flash all signs have disappeared. I cannot tell you how thrilled I am to have this under control and know how to manage it. Having had skin problems myself as a child, I really did not want Barnaby to go through what I went through so when we met Dr Harley, I knew we were onto a good thing! When we

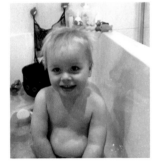

met he instantly connected with Barnaby and gave me every confidence as a parent that this was absolutely the right thing to be doing.

I have subsequently recommended Dr Harley to friends, whose children have varying forms of eczema and I cannot thank him enough for making the process so easy and successful. Anyone with eczema, young or old should speak to Dr Harley Farmer.

The next part is probably best presented as exerts from the emails between me and Dr Farmer as that shows how he interacts.

Phili: I've developed bl**dy eczema on my hands...... Why? How? What out of all the lotions and potions I have for Barnaby what can I try?! He's running around with baby soft skin, looking lovely and I'm here with scabby, scaly hands! Honestly, his skin is so much better, I hardly even put foam emollient on him now - AMAZING!

No idea why I've got it on my hands as I've actually never had it on my hands. Can it be hormonal as I'm pregnant again and I was just wondering if that may have caused it?

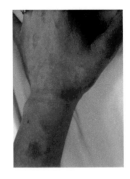

Dr Harley: First, congratulations on your pregnancy. On the basis of the photos (of your hands), it looks as though you need to regain a proper balance in those red patches of skin. The redness and resulting itch are the appropriate reaction to something and we need to find and remove that something. ... Use the foam emollient as your only skin wash for a while and also apply it as an emollient when your hands are dry. ... You will have extra stresses from your pregnancy and life in general. I'm told being a Mum is a hectic job! Take a moment to appreciate the wonders of being able to be a Mum of such a wonderful little boy and the joys of anticipation for the next child. Yes, it's hectic. Yet it's also wonderful and rewarding. You will want to be in balance for them both, the rest of your family and yourself. You need to remember yourself. There won't be anything "wrong" and we just want to regain the balance. My task is to help you find that balance.

Phili: I think it's safe to say Barnaby and my skin are clearly lovers of the foam emollient.... Hands are heaps better, not perfect yet but SO much better, so thank you. I'm convinced it must be hormone related to this pregnancy, I've had all sorts of 'skin issues' this time round that I've never had before! If you ever fancied

developing something for nappy rash I'd be in on that, blimey Barnaby has really suffered over the last month or so, no idea why.

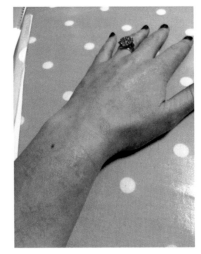

Dr Harley: That's great Phili. Or at least it was until the nappy rash part!

Phili: New hand attached!!!! ... You'll be pleased to hear that I've actually self diagnosed a good remedy for nappy rash 'foam emollient' ..... So should people ask you... It works!

As always I appreciate your help and I'm

forever telling people to talk to you as soon as I hear the word eczema!
Thanks again
Phili

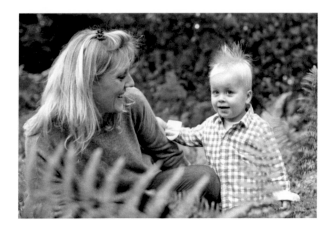

CHAPTER 7

A second-level disease

At the beginning of this book I presented some definitions of eczema. You will recall how conflicting and confusing they were. Someone with eczema can also develop new skin rashes that have nothing to do with their eczema. They are just skin rashes similar to those seen on people who have never had eczema. Yet those rashes on the eczema sufferer's skin add to the confusion. Are they part of the eczema or just rashes? Regardless of that distinction, emollients and moisturisers will probably be put all over their skin anyway to "*manage the eczema*" even if they are enjoying a phase of no eczema. So does it really matter what the new red patches of skin actually are? Yes, it does.

A practical way of explaining why it matters is to imagine a parent whose child is in a period of remission from eczema. At the time, the child's skin looks normal and healthy. Then the child develops a skin rash and the parent takes the child to their family doctor. The parent might tell the doctor one of two things:

1. my child has an eczema flare-up
2. my child has a skin rash.

Can you see how the choice of statement might take the doctor's thinking down completely different routes? If the parent mentions eczema and the doctor is thinking eczema, the advice will be to apply emollients to the red areas on the assumption that the skin redness is eczema. In complete contrast, if the doctor is thinking skin rash, it's quite likely the advice could centre on the many factors that can cause skin rashes in any child. That's still a very broad and challenging topic yet most people find it easier to have a practical discussion on skin rashes and the probable causes than they do on eczema.

For statement 1 the medical advice is likely to involve emollients. For statement 2 there's a fair chance the advice could include factors like adverse reactions to foods.

Obviously the new rash may be the first sign of eczema coming back. But what if it isn't?

This is really important. If the child is prescribed emollients, the parent will apply those foreign products to the rash. As you know, there will be skin cracks in the rash. Some of the emollient will find its way down those cracks and when it's detected by the immune system, there will be inflammation in an attempt to expel that foreign emollient from within the skin. If more emollient is then applied, as usually happens, the child will enter a cycle where the product used to manage the rash will be the cause of subsequent inflammation. Once this cycle has begun, the product will be maintaining the skin inflammation, the dermatitis. That's why I introduced the phrase Product Maintained Dermatitis.

How can this be used in the battle against eczema? By distinguishing between skin rashes and eczema. If you're preparing to argue that they're the same thing, please trust me a while longer and read on a little more. As it happens you are right but there is advantage to be gained in forcing a distinction. There are times when a new rash is not eczema and I will concentrate on that for now.

I would like you to envisage eczema as a second-level condition with a skin rash being the first level. For some people that is easiest to visualise in words. For others, it's best put in a diagram. To cover both groups I will use words first followed by a diagram.

The base level is normal healthy skin. It steps up one level to a skin rash. This is not eczema; it is just the sort of skin rash any person with normal healthy skin might have. If products which are foreign to the human body are applied to that rash, some of the product can go down skin cracks inducing new inflammation. That elevates it to the second level, eczema. Since there is so much confusion associated with that word 'eczema' try replacing the word with the phrase Product Maintained Dermatitis or PMD. Remember, this second level happened when product applied to the skin rash (first level) went IN the skin leading to inflammation against the product. When more product is added the product will keep the inflammation going. That is product maintained dermatitis which is the second level or eczema.

If you stop applying the product, there is nothing to maintain the dermatitis and the inflammation goes. The skin 'steps down' from the second level. If the cause of the original rash is still there, the rash will still be there. However if the cause of the rash is gone and the underlying rash is no longer there, stopping the application of product will allow the skin to step all the way down to normal skin.

That is what happens in most eczema sufferers when the product which was maintaining the dermatitis is no longer applied. If that product is not going down skin cracks inducing inflammation, there is nothing for the immune system to expel so there is no need for inflammation. The skin goes direct from second-level condition to normal skin.

Now for the diagram.

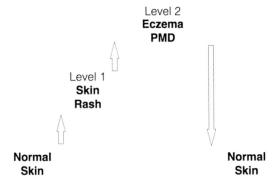

In summary, a new skin rash is the first level. When product applied to that rash induces new inflammation, that is the second level.

Recall how eczema sufferers are advised to apply products all over their skin, even the areas that are not affected by eczema.

Now consider a situation where someone with a history of eczema does develop a new patch of red skin rash which is just a normal skin rash and not related to eczema. The emollient they are told to apply all over themselves will find its way down skin cracks in that new rash leading to inflammation. The rash (first level) will become eczema (second level) *because* the product has induced new inflammation. Further application of the product to *manage* the inflammation will *maintain* the inflammation.

That is **Product Maintained Dermatitis**. That's when *manage* means *maintain*.

Now return your mind to that child who develops a skin rash at a time when they no longer had eczema. If the doctor's thinking is automatically directed towards eczema the child will have emollients applied to the rash. That can cause eczema, even though the rash may have been completely unrelated to eczema. The thinking leads to the diagnosis. The thought of it possibly being eczema becomes a self-fulfilling prophecy. When eczema is caused by the treatment, the original thought that it may have been eczema is confirmed. That's a terrible shame if it was just a simple skin rash that was temporary and about to go away. That is what I call the **eczema trap** where the disease is caused and then maintained by the treatment.

In contrast, if the doctor was thinking of other causes that may have led to the new skin rash, the parent could be advised to consider things like diet. If no product is applied to the new rash and the cause of the rash is discovered and eliminated, the rash will go away. The child will not become caught in the eczema trap.

Now I would like to present a personal story of an adult. That adult is me. I had bad eczema when I was a young man at university and during the early stages of my research career. As my knowledge developed, especially in relation to the way our immune system reacts in skin disease, I found a way to end my eczema. However I was still me and my skin was still my skin. I still had the sensitive skin which led me into eczema in the first place.

In recent years I've found having sensitive skin very useful. I now have a company where we create very gentle skin cleansing products. Those products are intended for use by all people, including those with a tendency for eczema and the rest who have normal healthy skin; people of every ethnic group and age. I always test new products on myself before anyone else is asked to try them. The reason is that my sensitive skin allows me to establish how my skin reacts to each new formulation. My technical knowledge gained during a long career in successfully ending diseases allows me to 'visualise' what is happening on and in my skin when a new formulation is applied.

That means I can use my very sensitive skin to ensure the products are correct for people with normal skin.

When I want to ensure the new products are suitable for people with eczema, which is far more challenging, my very sensitive skin becomes invaluable. I just apply one of the well known branded moisturisers or emollients to my sensitive skin knowing it will cause eczema within a week. I then stop using the branded product and switch to the new cleansing product I want to test. If the eczema goes away, I know the new test product does NOT maintain the dermatitis. It is then shared with others within my circle who share my values and, in due course, it is offered to the market.

The vital message of this story is that I can turn what appears to be normal skin into eczema in a week by using readily available skincare products. Consider what that means for other people who happen to develop dry skin and opt to use a well known branded moisturiser. For some of them, the product will lead to eczema. The product leads to Product Maintained Dermatitis.

The thing most people don't know, which you do, is that normal appearing skin can have skin cracks. If applying products does not lead to inflammation you know the products did not go deep enough down the cracks to be detected by the immune system. However, if the immune system reacts with inflammation, you know the product did go deep enough to induce inflammation. What happens next depends on whether the person applies more product to the inflamed skin. If they do, they have Product Maintained Dermatitis; eczema. If they don't, they don't.

Now consider a person who has been free of eczema for some time, a person who appreciates that eczema is a second-level condition. The next time they develop a skin rash, they know why they should NOT apply products which might go into their skin and induce inflammation turning the rash into eczema. When they forget, as sometimes happens, they recognise the eczema for what it is, a second-level issue, and stop using the product. The skin then heals itself by expelling the product. The skin can do that because the chemical insult is no longer being applied.

That is the value of distinguishing between skin rashes, which are just rashes, and eczema which is product maintained dermatitis. For readers with a thorough technical knowledge of all types of eczema, please appreciate this is mainly referring to *atopic* eczema. However, when you use this logic to other forms of eczema you may find it very useful. Sufferers of other forms of eczema who used this logic to end their eczema became EXeczema successes.

This clue allows people to end their eczema and prevent it coming back.

If you find this confusing, please go back and read this chapter again as the understanding of this fundamental clue is essential before proceeding.

If you accept this concept of eczema being a second-level condition, you are two thirds of the way to having all the clues. Even though there have been a lot of words used, the two clues are still very simple, aren't they?

1. Whether a product is ON the skin or IN the skin makes a huge difference.
2. Eczema is a second-level condition.

EXeczema® Success

Rajveer's Journey

When I heard of the NewGenn company to be honest it took a few weeks for me to come round to the idea of trying something new. I thought to myself how can

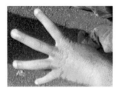

eczema possibly be cured in 2 weeks, but then I read the book and everything just seemed to make sense. Rajveer had eczema from the age of six months and has had followup appointments every six months. On every appointment there just seemed to be the same outcome that I am doing well with the steroids and creams, but in my eyes Rajveer's skin was in a very bad state.

He didn't have breaks in between eczema flare ups; his skin was always sore and irritated. This has led to 2 hospital admissions with strong antibiotics and antivirals to mend his skin.

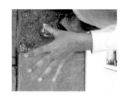

I couldn't believe that I did not need these steroids or creams as they were doing more harm than any good. Once I started using the hand rub and wipes, although Rajveer's skin went completely dry and flaky after the first week, I could see that his skin was no longer red. By the end of the 2nd week I was convinced that this treatment has worked.

We are now over 2 months into the treatment and although I use the wipes and hand rub from time to time Rajveer no longer has eczema. Gone are the nights of interrupted sleep from scratching.

I am glad I tried the treatment because it really does work. To any parent who has a child with eczema I would definitely recommend they try it but not before reading the book because they will not give their 100% commitment as they won't understand the program."

Nicki Rooprai, UK

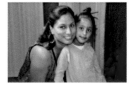

CHAPTER 8

28 day generation time for skin cells

You've reached the third and final clue, and the best time for me to explain how I became involved in ending eczema in children. I happily admit it was accidental. I did not set out to do it! After all, it was well known that you can't cure eczema so why waste valuable time trying? Sad, isn't it?

In association with infection control teams in British hospitals, I helped develop a set of hand hygiene products for nurses. The new products left a lovely feeling on their skin so some of the nurses took the products home to wash their children. I then began receiving phone calls with the mothers, the nurses, saying "Dr Harley, thank you for curing my child's eczema". You can imagine my surprise as I was not working with children at the time. However the products *were* proving very effective at ending the dermatitis which is so common on nurses' hands. That is now called Chronic Hand Eczema so I was already ending one form of eczema; in adults. It was conceivable that I had unintentionally developed a means of ending atopic eczema in children.

I was acutely aware of the prevailing belief that "eczema can't be cured". I knew my own eczema had gone away and I'd been free of eczema for decades. Did this new accidental finding in children suggest it was worth challenging the established paradigm that eczema can't be cured? I definitely thought so. The eczema had undoubtedly ended but would it stay away? Was it simply a coincidence in which each child was about to end the eczema anyway and my products just happened to be there at the time? Nobody could answer those questions and obviously I was not going to cause eczema in the children again just so I could see it go away.

I chose to seize the opportunity to investigate further. I looked at the ingredients in the products which had been applied to the children prior to my products being used. Many of the previous products contained high levels of mineral oil, a major ingredient in many moisturisers, creams, lotions and emollients. I knew those chemicals were brilliant at provoking the immune system, inducing inflammation in a valid attempt to expel the foreign chemical. It became an easy matter of asking whether the provocative chemical could be detected by the immune system when those products were used to *manage* eczema? That question was very easily answered and you know why.

The next step was to ask the mothers how soon the skin redness disappeared after they began using our products; how soon after they *stopped* using the previous products? The average answer was 14 days.

I knew the skin replaces itself every month. Every day we all shed dead skin cells from the outside of our skin and for each cell that's shed, a new one is created on the inside to replace it. We all have a constant outward flow of skin cells and it takes each cell a month to reach the outside and fall off. So if our products were having a positive effect in 14 days, that was happening well within the generation time for skin cells.

It occurred to me that we might have simply replaced products which 'provoked' the immune system with products that did not provoke. I knew the products I'd developed for nurses' hands contained an absolute minimum of chemical. In fact they all contained around 99% water as I designed them to cleanse the skin and water is good for that. They had excellent antibacterial properties and they left a lovely feeling on skin, but their primary function was to cleanse the skin. Could it be possible the tiny level of ingredients was simply so low it did not warrant action by the immune system? If so, the next generation of skin cells would all reach the outside and make normal healthy skin, even in the presence of our very watery products.

Could it have possibly been that simple? Even I was skeptical saying "surely not". After all, eczema was such a complicated disease with all sorts of unexplained things going on. It would almost be disrespectful to all those people suffering prolonged misery to believe the eczema could be ended with such simplicity. So I fought my instincts and romantic nature for some time in an attempt to find the complications I must have been missing. I really gave it a good shot and was left with a simple answer. Yes, it really is that easy. If you stop causing eczema the skin heals itself.

Now you can better appreciate why I avoid offering judgement and criticism to those who are skeptical about the good story presented here. Even I chose to disbelieve until I had looked at every angle, so I respect their feelings. I still do. Every new person who ventures onto the EXeczema journey leaves me wondering if we have the right story for that individual. Can it be as simple for them too? The benefit of remaining so skeptical, despite having so many people endorse the logic, is that we remain open to new clues. There are many millions of people around the world who still have eczema which equates to millions of clues we have yet to collect, scrutinise and share. Perhaps I will grow out of this inherent skepticism in time but if that meant closing the way for new clues, then I would prefer to stay as I am. Open to new knowledge. Forever listening.

Here I will instil an element of caution. Simply going "cold turkey" and just stopping the use of the old immune-provoking products leads to other skin issues. That goes a long way to explaining the syndrome people call "Steroid Withdrawal". I'll say very little about it here other than I believe those afflicted by that condition can find useful clues in this book.

Returning to eczema, the best improvement comes by taking time. Be gentle with the damaged skin. Over several days there must be a transition, a gradual replacement of the previous immune-provoking products with ones the immune system ignores.

The new products must also:

1. contain a very low level of chemical content
2. be excellent at cleansing skin
3. have the appropriate level of antibacterial action
4. be very gentle on new skin
5. have no irritating properties and
6. be safe for even the broken skin of tiny babies.

Products with that many attributes are rarely subtle; they tend to need a range of chemicals in order to satisfy each attribute resulting in the final products being provocative. It seems subtlety and minimalism had low priority for those developing the previous products.

Why is this relevant in ending eczema? My new phrase of Product Maintained Dermatitis provides the clue. As you know, it takes a month for each skin cell to reach the outside and complete its life cycle.

In healthy skin, each outwardly migrating skin cell plays its individual part in supplying the components which make up the skin barrier. Healthy skin has a healthy skin barrier just below the surface, and that skin barrier allows just the right amount of water to move outwards to keep the skin in water balance. Of equal importance, the healthy skin barrier also prevents chemical irritants moving into the skin.

In patches of inflamed skin, the new skin cells are still moving outwards but the inflammation stops them making the components needed to make a healthy skin barrier. When the skin barrier is defective, chemicals can enter the skin. The more intense the inflammation, the more chemical can enter the skin.

Now combine the month-long generation time and the negative effect of inflammation on the skin barrier.

If you have been applying a product to eczema **for over a month** and the eczema is still there, begin assuming that product is involved in maintaining the dermatitis. That product is provoking the immune system into using inflammation to expel the product from IN the skin.

That product is *part of the problem* if the immune system is reacting against it. *Part of the solution* is to stop applying that product.

It is the same regardless of whether the product is 'natural' or 'organic' or 'green' or has a globally trusted brand name or was prescribed by a doctor. If you have been applying the product for over a month and the eczema is still there, the product is involved with the inflammation. If the immune system does not like it, that's a very useful clue, wouldn't you agree? The person who sold it to you may like it, but now that you are 'listening' to the skin and the immune system, where would you prefer to place your trust? If you have been using the product for over a month and the eczema is still there, you have enough information to make a choice. Keep using the same product and watch the skin keep reacting with inflammation, or stop using the product so the skin no longer needs to react against it.

If the skin doesn't like it the skin doesn't like it. Few things could be simpler than that.

You now have all three clues. Would you like a way of challenging the sheer simplicity? Remember,

1. You know it makes a huge difference whether a product is ON the skin or IN the skin.
2. You understand why it helps so much to view eczema as a second-level condition.
3. And you know skin replaces itself every month.

Now bring all three clues together to help with this challenge. Ask yourself whether the same product was inducing inflammation in the non-eczema areas of skin? No, it wasn't. Therefore the problem only occurs in areas of damaged skin where we know the product can go IN the skin deep enough for the immune system to detect it and be provoked into inflammation.

Therefore the product will be fine on a person with normal healthy skin, just as it's fine on a healthy area of skin on an eczema sufferer.

This is vitally important so it's equally important that you challenge it in your mind. In the path metaphor, step off the path for a moment and really, really, challenge this concept.

- You are in control now,
- you have all three clues,
- you know others have done really well by stepping off the path to examine things more intently,
- you have the confidence from seeing others who've chosen to do the same.

Could something else have been maintaining the dermatitis; the inflammation; the eczema?

1. There was nothing 'wrong' with the patient's ability to make healthy skin as they were making perfectly normal skin in their non-eczema areas.
2. The children in whom this simplicity was first revealed developed normal skin in half the generation time of skin cells. So the next generation of cells moving outwards were capable of making normal skin when the reason for the inflammation was removed.

3. Immune-suppressing drugs like steroids were not needed to stop the inflammation. The inflammation disappeared automatically once the immune-provoking products were no longer within the skin.

4. There was nothing 'wrong' with the immune system since it settled down as soon as the provocative products were gone. The inflammation went when those products went. The inflammation was not *atopic* if it can be explained this easily; if it was the appropriate and proportionate response to a chemical insult.

5. Cleansing products made almost entirely of water did not provoke the immune system.

6. The skin healed itself without any need for specific healing-enhancing technology.

Unless I'm missing something, the previous products used on those children were the only thing that could have been causing the immune system to react with inflammation in their skin. That means those provocative products were causing the Product Maintained Dermatitis, the eczema.

Does the relevance of the skin replacing itself every month and its association with Product Maintained Dermatitis rest easily with you? If not, please go back and read this chapter again as the understanding of this fundamental clue is essential before proceeding.

You now know all of the three clues and you've tested the relevance of your new knowledge to eczema.

You control the three pieces of this jigsaw. Three-piece jigsaws are quite simple, aren't they? When you put those three pieces together, does the whole imbalance called eczema make sense? Good, now let's extend the jigsaw analogy. Prior to this moment, were you trying to make a plausible picture out of pieces from multiple jigsaws? You had pieces from the psychology jigsaw, the inflammation jigsaw, the hereditary jigsaw, the product jigsaw, the parenting jigsaw and many more. Completing a huge jigsaw is hard enough when you have pieces from only one jigsaw. Are you happy to accept how hard it is to complete a complicated jigsaw when you are given pieces from many jigsaws all mixed together? If so, are you ready to see why I don't suggest judgement for those still attempting to find one picture among many?

You appreciate now why it helps to let others come to their own realisations in their own time. Let them see why it has been so hard for them to end eczema when their resources are in the same muddled confusing format you faced before reading this book.

Is this the first time you have had eczema explained this way? If so, take a moment to wonder what that means. Really give yourself time for this one.

Do you appreciate what you can now achieve; why you can end eczema and prevent it coming back?

That's right. If you like to use the word "cure" that's entirely up to you. You are in control of eczema now so it's your choice. You might find the word cure provokes undue reactions from people who insist that "eczema can't be cured". Rather than entering a heated debate, it might be easier to point out that when there is nothing to maintain the eczema, the skin simply heals itself. No cure is actually needed.

Before proceeding to explain the EXeczema® programme, it's best to have a very brief review of how the three clues work together within that programme.

- You now appreciate that products ON the skin have little relevance whereas products which go IN and provoke the immune system will result in inflammation in the skin.
- You also know that putting those products onto reddened skin has the strong potential to induce Product Maintained Dermatitis, also known as eczema.
- Any products that have been put on eczema for over a month should be considered to be maintaining the eczema.

What are the useful consequences of that new knowledge?

1. First, this knowledge set is probably new to you. Therefore any bad experiences from previous attempts to end eczema can be set aside as you did not have this knowledge to help you at that time. Past failures can be left in the past.
2. You want to stop using the previous products as soon as practical; all those products which you can associate with eczema; products that have been maintaining the eczema.

3. You will require new skincare products which do not provoke the immune system; products that will cleanse the skin gently while the skin is healing itself from the inside outwards.

4. Your confidence in knowing how to end eczema and prevent it coming back provides the boost you want to succeed.

5. At any time you may want to take some time to gather more confidence before proceeding to end the eczema.

6. Your rate of progress to EXeczema is entirely your choice.

7. You are in control. The outcome is up to you.

8. When the eczema is gone and you have confidence that your new knowledge will prevent the eczema coming back, you can 'give back' to society. You'll be able to help others achieve the same health and happiness in a life after eczema.

I hope you'll agree that's an impressive list. Putting you in control of eczema is one of the most liberating joys in the whole global EXeczema® campaign. That is just as appropriate regardless of whether you are:

i.   a doctor or other healthcare professional providing positive advice to patients knowing they can now end their eczema,

ii. a parent able to free your child from the misery of the eczema trap,

iii. an eczema sufferer who has now realised you can end the disease and get your life back,

iv. an education professional who can now guide eczema sufferers to this knowledge to end the imbalance so it's not there to affect exam results,

v.   a friend who really wants to help someone important to you gain the health and happiness available from ending eczema.

Many others have achieved success and ended eczema which is why this book can be based on so many wonderful comments from those who've chosen to give back by sharing their joyful experiences.

EXeczema® Success

Adrian Smith

I've had eczema and dermatitis all of my life, with too many flare-ups to count, including one as a student when I was hospitalised to bring it under control.

As a child my eczema was in the usual places; elbow, backs of knees, but as an adult it moved to become much more visible on my face, scalp and hands.

My management regime has always been based around steroids of different potency and a lifetime of experimenting with emollients, from large pots of grease to small tubs of expensive moisturiser.

Eventually I found products that seemed to suit me, but the flare-ups still came, particularly in the winter months and during periods of stress. I couldn't imagine facing the day without emollients.

So when Harley first advised me that the emollients could be the problem and recommended I stop them entirely, I wasn't just sceptical, I was somewhat offended — and very defensive.

I had never really questioned the logic before, but Harley's book politely challenged my beliefs and presented a positive view beyond my boundaries. The more I thought about what the innocuous-looking white emollient is made of and the reactions I have to it, the more sense Harley's advice made.

Harley's insight proved to be a turning point. My dermatitis cleared up quickly and though extremely dry, particularly initially, my skin was much calmer as it was given a break to do its job without battling emollient for the first time in years.

My skin is now infinitely better and more manageable, with long periods when eczema is not an issue. The ongoing challenge for me is managing my stress, allergy triggers and finding essential but potentially irritating products such as sun creams that suit my skin.

For the first time in my life, I'm in control of my skin.

Harley has worked wonders on my eczema and I will always be very grateful to him for his knowledge and support.

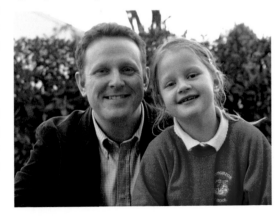

CHAPTER 9

The EXeczema® programme

The most wonderful aspect of the EXeczema programme is the way those who succeed in ending eczema provide comments which allow us to continually improve the programme.

Years ago I ended my own eczema and limited my activities to helping the few people who knew of my success. Over time the concept grew as I learned from helping others with their limiting beliefs and personal boundaries. Whenever the trend became more widely known, I was met with anything from ridicule for believing in such romantic success to downright condemnation for letting people think they could ever succeed in escaping eczema.

I found that negative response ironic since most people grow out of eczema, proving that eczema is not the natural state. *Ending* eczema is the *natural* state. That suggests eczema is simply a lack of balance in parts of the skin. I knew how devastating it was in certain individuals yet their affliction was simply the same lack of balance at a much greater magnitude.

My training in physiology and pathology means I can interpret the skin changes. The training I gained in achieving a PhD in preventing diseases helps me study the medical and scientific literature to gather clues. All my life I've been keen to know how things progress; what starts them, why they keep going, what the end is. As I earned more qualifications, it became obvious that my main passion lies in what they call pathogenesis — the way disease progresses. My most recent training and qualification were in psychology to satisfy my interest in why some people stay with a disease, despite knowing how to end it, and why others actively grasp the opportunity the moment they see it.

From the perspective of that lifelong quest for knowledge and understanding, the various steps on the path to EXeczema are obvious to me. This book and the EXeczema programme are my way of presenting it all to everyone so those who choose to can improve it for others.

I created the new word EXeczema to mean the time *after* eczema. The concept arose from my utilisation of psychology in guiding people who were ready to end their eczema but didn't know how to begin. The advice and information they had been able to find elsewhere was negative and reinforced the limiting belief that you can't cure eczema. If there is nowhere to go, it's hard to begin, wouldn't you agree?

That word "cure" had a lot of associations, most of which were distinctly unhelpful.

My new word EXeczema enables me to say "I don't do eczema. I do the time *after* eczema". Those of you with psychology experience will recognise the relevance. Discussions about eczema focus on eczema. There are many millions of people taking part in eczema discussions around the world. Despite all their words and combined effort, there are still many, many, millions of people with eczema, the vast majority of whom have come to accept that you can't cure eczema. In essence, all those words used in the eczema debate offer no choice but eczema. The effect of "doing eczema" is you keep doing it!

I felt it would be helpful to find a way of introducing "no eczema" into the available choices. The time after eczema is the best way to do it as that provides a target for someone who wants to move on from eczema. It allows an achievable end point; a distinct goal. I'm always extremely careful to avoid any suggestion of the time between eczema and EXeczema as I want people to be in control of their own journey, especially the speed with which they reach that time *after* eczema.

Control and freedom to choose are two things I find those who only discuss eczema seem to lack. Some people do not want those options as they firmly believe there can be no choice other than remaining as they are, in the state of imbalance. If that is their belief they will prove themselves right.

I choose to focus on the people who are seeking new choices. They're the early adopters who are effectively pre-selecting themselves. They tend to be the people who are excited by change and like providing comments to enhance the journey for those following. Their suggestions fill the gap between eczema and my vision of EXeczema and this book reflects their views and comments.

Positioning a person's thoughts in a time after eczema enables them to leave the previous debate behind and relocate themselves at their point of success. In their mind, during that exercise, the eczema is gone. They are then schooled in how to look back at their barriers from the viewpoint of having achieved their goal. As expected, all the barriers which had kept them constrained look completely different when viewed from the perspective of having overcome them. The value lies in the people seeing their own solutions to each of their barriers, revealing choices they could not see before.

The person still has to take action and follow the path to success. The gain comes from them coming to their own realisation that success is one of their available choices. Success is permissible, possible and achievable. They realise they are *allowed* to end eczema.

Reactions to a new concept like EXeczema follow a well established trend. First comes a vision, an idea in someone's mind; in this case, mine. Then the vision is given a useable and memorable title, the new word EXeczema. The novelty attracts early adopters to give it a try. Success prompts them to comment, easing the path for those who come next; the main population, whose confidence arises from seeing success. The last group are those who opt never to venture onto the path to freedom from eczema and they have perfectly valid reasons for selecting that choice.

The EXeczema programme is intentionally left to evolve as we learn more. Each person who travels the path earns the right to contribute their views on how to improve the journey for those who follow. It's fantastic to realise we have a huge number of early adopters among the many millions of people around the world who still have eczema. Most of them have yet to hear of the programme and as more of them do, the early adopters among them will react like the previous early adopters. Put very simply, they will do their journey their way as that's who they are. Early adopters rarely do as they are told which is fortunate as they are happy to self-test their own new ideas and provide comments. Since I am always listening, they provide new ways of improving the process.

The first wave of early adopters were instrumental in helping me conceive the EXeczema concept. The next wave led to making it more tangible to a wider audience. Those in each new wave test the programme as it is when they first meet it and their comments bring enhancements. It's humbling to realise how many people wanted to help and further enhance the EXeczema programme. As the team grows and new early adopters do what they do, we all gain from the privilege of being given their personal contributions. To an early adopter, the excitement derives from doing something the moment they become aware of it, regardless of whether others have been along the path before them.

The reason I leave the programme in such a progressive fluid state lies in my level of knowledge. Many people tell me I know so much; I graciously accept their complements and quietly remind myself how much I have yet to learn. This keeps me open to suggestions. I genuinely believe eczema can become a rare event; we can end existing eczema and prevent new eczema. That combination of humility and will means the EXeczema programme is much bigger than me. It arose in my positive, free-thinking, mind. Yet the real beauty lies in how it allows so many others to reach a goal they come to realise is practical and plausible. You *can* end eczema.

My thrill comes in knowing many millions of people will encompass the EXeczema concept, even though that will still leave millions around the world with imbalanced skin. I'm writing this in England where we currently have about six million eczema sufferers. Therefore use of the word "millions" is easily justified. Extrapolating that around the world shows just how many millions of sufferers exist. I have a romantic notion that every person who achieves EXeczema success is another person who might provide the gem of an idea which will ignite interest in those I have yet to reach. It's my way of leading people by letting them see a better option. If they like the new option they will come to their own realisations and join me in the place and time called EXeczema. I will be helping them gain health and happiness.

The last few pages have been very much in the field of

psychology. To many readers that future goal is a bit intangible making it a challenge to visualise taking their first step on the journey. Is there a way of providing greater clarity and a more accessible view of where they are, stuck in the eczema imbalance state? Yes, and it relates to the products they have been using on the eczematous skin.

Almost all the emollients and moisturisers available around the world are creams, ointments or lotions. The chemical ingredients mean the products are opaque; you can't see through them. That's partly because they have a very high level of chemical content. As you know, most of the chemicals they contain, except water, are foreign to the human body so the more foreign chemical there is, the more chance there is of it going IN the skin provoking the immune system to inflammation and eczema.

Opacity becomes a word worth focusing your thoughts on. The opaque products containing all those chemicals at high levels have been used for decades while the number of eczema cases was increasing around the world. Since I was seeking a way of reducing the incidence of eczema, there was logic in looking at the opposite of high chemical levels. Was it possible to serve the needs and wants of users by going to the other extreme and having an absolute minimum of chemical content? Of course it was, if you were content to be seen as separate from the pack. Few people seek to be different, but if you are aiming to create a different outcome it makes sense to offer something different. What would a product with the *absolute minimum* of chemical content look like, especially if it contained none of the mineral oil type of foreign chemicals? Such a product would be transparent, clear. **Clarity** becomes the key word.

That presents you with another choice, this time between opacity and clarity. Opacity came from the products which were used to manage eczema; you can associate opacity with eczema. Clarity comes with the products used by those who are now EXeczema successes. You can associate clarity with the time after eczema.

Now consider how those words opacity and clarity are also used to describe how well we understand a topic. Opacity means the thinking is confused; it usually leads to more of the same. Clarity allows the best path to be seen leading to change for the better.

I invite the reader to take this pivotal moment to advance from opacity and embrace clarity. That goes for both the products used on the skin and the thinking process. Would you agree that opacity has not served eczema sufferers well while clarity makes the goal easier to visualise and achieve?

It is now appropriate to discuss the actual EXeczema® programme. In this text I will use the names of specific products created in my company in order to explain the process. There will almost certainly be other brands which achieve the same but because I could not find any it became necessary to create these. It seems very few people make skincare products based on clarity, possibly because the thinking which leads to simplicity appears to be a scarce resource. Achieving more with less requires a rare skill.

The EXeczema programme is a series of steps. It will evolve with time as more people provide suggestions so please visit www.execzema.org for the current version if you are reading this book some time after the publication date of **February 2016**.

The best results come from following the steps in the sequence described in the EXeczema Instructions document you have downloaded.

You are now in the beautiful situation of being able to share your experiences. Share the joy of clarity in thought and product. Do you remember what it was like when you had neither? Great. That is the feeling of despair and hopelessness you can now alleviate in others.

There will be plenty of people who are still within the eczema trap and you now have the privilege of being able to help them. Do remember that nobody *pushed you* to EXeczema success; you came to your own realisations on being shown the option of ending eczema. You chose to examine the 3 clues, learn the new knowledge, select your preferred speed, perhaps chose to take a while at the side of the path and then proceeded to the end goal. When you are helping someone else match your success, give them the same degree of freedom to choose. Most will follow your path, the one you reveal to them through clarity. Congratulations, you have chosen to give back. It's a wonderful feeling.

Some will refuse your offer. Be ready for that; it's fine. If you give them time they may follow later. If not, they have chosen to stay in the state of eczema imbalance for their own reason. Respect their choice and realise you can help best by simply letting them watch others complete the path to freedom from eczema.

That is the EXeczema® programme. Simplicity and clarity.

EXeczema® Success

Beryl – young enough to learn new tricks

Written by her daughter Joan.

A few months ago, if I had come across the EXeczema website, I probably would have assumed that this was yet another site set up with YET another way to treat eczema — which no doubt would be unsuccessful. I had spent hours over the past years surfing the Internet for a solution to ending my mother's eczema.

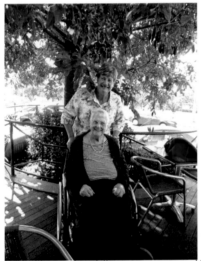

Occasionally I found something which helped but the eczema always returned, very red, raw and itchy — no better. It was the same story with treatments advised by doctors, including those involved with treating her other health ailments during long, extended hospital stays. I had come to believe that the eczema was just something she had to live with — for life!

Then, how fortunate we were to have met Dr Harley Farmer, founder of the EXeczema programme. He was in Australia at the time and was introduced by someone we trust. He kindly offered to talk with us about the programme. He genuinely appeared to believe that his programme could 'stop' the eczema and that it would NOT return ….. But firstly, he wanted us to understand the Science behind what had been happening to my mother's skin and the reason for the resulting eczema with which she had been living for years ….. and his explanation made complete sense!

After a short consultation with my mother we were on a mission, a mission to end her eczema. I would not have been willing to embrace the programme if she had not been serious about doing **exactly** as Dr Farmer suggested. There would be no cheating, *not even a little bit*. I felt that the process had to be followed exactly as he described to ensure that it would work.

I won't pretend it was easy. The medical world had effectively written my mother's eczema off so I didn't expect it to be easy. Many times my mother wanted to return to applying creams to stop the itching, those same creams that were causing the eczema. But she is 91 and is in a wheelchair. She was not able to reach down to apply those creams to here legs and feet. I was the person caring for her, her feet in particular, and I could see some improvement. I was not willing to give in to her pleases — not just yet. I continued with the bathing many times a day, and Dr Farmer had recently given me a bottle of his gel to prevent the itching. And it worked! From then on when my mother's legs and feet itched (mostly at night), I applied the gel and we got by.

Now the good news! The legs and feet look great! They are not fiery or itchy. We are no longer getting the breakouts. In fact, the eczema has GONE!

P.S. I wrote the above when my mother was younger!! She is now 94 and everything above is still relevant.

CHAPTER 10

The holistic person

The skin is an organ of the body, the biggest organ we have. It's the only organ you can easily see from the outside, making it an extremely useful tool for assessing what is going on inside. It's sometimes amazing to see how quickly the skin can react to a signal from another organ. Consider a person who blushes on hearing a delicate comment; the ears hear it, the brain interprets it and the skin goes red, all within seconds. A person is a whole being of which the skin is just one part.

Skin is our outer packaging. It keeps us in and the rest of the world out. That's a tough challenge which is one of the reasons the skin needs to replace itself so often; every month as you know. It's nature's way of ensuring our 'packaging' is kept in fresh working order.

Yet to live, we need our bodies to take in and pass out material. The body has three ways of taking material in:

1. the lungs when we breath in
2. the mouth when we swallow
3. and to a much lesser extent, the skin when it absorbs materials.

Our body has four ways of expelling material:
1. exhaled breath
2. faeces
3. urine
4. and skin secretions.

Therefore the skin holds us together, takes certain chemicals in and lets other chemicals out. A healthy person has healthy skin. They are in balance with their skin. Someone with unhealthy skin is out of balance.

I really like the concept of *balance* as it implies things aren't irretrievable when a person is just out of balance. There's still a chance; all is not lost, even if it does feel horrible. Most 'out of balance' things being reflected in the skin can be fixed as the skin is just revealing the whole person being out of balance with nature. When you take action to re-balance the person, their skin will reflect that new and better state.

Although skin is our packaging, it's a lot smarter than plastic wrapping. Cuts in skin bleed, clot, scab over and then heal. We've all witnessed it. It's automatic and our contribution is to let the skin get on with healing itself. No drug was needed to 'cure' the skin that was cut. When we choose to do things which upset that natural healing process, the skin can't heal itself in the optimal manner until we give the skin its chance to heal. We can interfere but the default of automatic healing just waits for us to 'stop being such a nuisance and get out of the way'. Then the skin heals.

A simple example is someone who picks at scabs, removing them. The skin will keep making new scabs as part of its automatic natural healing process. When the person finally stops removing the scabs, that healing process simply goes on to complete the healing. Normal healthy skin is just a matter of days away when the abuse stops. In really chronic cases where the scab has been repeatedly removed for a very long time, scarring of the skin may be the end result. That's still a natural healing process even though it leaves a permanent sign in the skin; a reminder of how detrimental the prolonged abuse was.

I like to suggest the skin is very *patient* packaging. When we decide to prevent the skin being normal and healthy, it will heal itself as far as we allow it and stop at the point where we stop it. As soon as we remove the barrier to healing, the skin immediately proceeds to complete the rest of the healing steps. Skin will wait. All is not lost in chronic eczema where the skin is being prevented from healing itself. Some of the EXeczema successes now have healthy normal skin after 70 years of unintentionally impeding their skin's route to healing itself. When those barriers were finally taken away, the healing process went to completion. Yes, there was some scarring on their healed skin, yet I feel the real scars were in their minds with the realisation of how the advice they were receiving for all those decades was just keeping them in misery. There is hope; help the skin help the person and amazing things happen.

The overall holistic discussion encompasses many aspects. A few of them are discussed in this chapter, although you will appreciate a lot more could be written on each one. In fact, entire books have been written about most of them. The objective here is to mention them in context to add validity to the reason why people aiming to end eczema can benefit so much from considering the whole person.

Chemical ingression

The outer layer of the skin is called the epidermis. On the inner edge of that layer new skin cells are made every day and they pass outwards to fall off eventually as dead, dried up, flakes. We don't see the vast majority of these tiny cells as they leave the surface. It's all done in beautiful balance without us needing to be aware.

Part way through their journey skin cells develop granules which collectively make up the skin barrier which controls the rate of water loss through the skin. If there are tiny invisible cracks in the epidermis, the cracks can extend though the skin barrier decreasing its ability to control outward water flow. Then more water is lost than should be the case. Where excess water can get out, other chemicals can get in and you know the relevance of that with eczema.

These tiny invisible cracks are the first indication that the skin is going to become dry. The cracks appear *before* a person senses dry skin. Therefore, by the time someone feels they have a dry patch of skin, they already have gaps in their skin defences which chemicals and products like opaque moisturisers can penetrate to induce inflammation.

That represents a state of imbalance. Applying opaque moisturisers to skin in this extra-permeable state can lead to inflammation and progress to eczema.

In relation to the holistic person, it is the mind that says the skin feels dry. It's the mind that decides which product should be put on dry patches of skin. In the context of managing eczema, the mind is doing things that put the skin into a greater state of imbalance. The skin will keep trying to heal itself but the mind's decision to use products which provoke the immune system into inflammation will retard the healing process. That's imbalance within the person. The mind can be helped with the set of 3 clues presented in this book. Once the mind has that and knows how to use it to best advantage, the mind can select clear skincare products which do not provoke the immune system. The skin dryness can then be overcome without inducing inflammation.

Genetic changes

Appreciating the wonders of skin is an essential part of understanding eczema. Almost every person with eczema has some parts of their skin which are not inflamed. That's important as it shows they are *capable* of making normal healthy skin. There is nothing 'wrong' with their skin, their immune system or the person.

Yet we are seeing an increasing number of tests done with the intention of finding genetic defects in individuals with eczema. There is no doubt that a very small proportion of people who have an absence of the filaggrin gene cannot make the granules in skin cells which other people use to create a proper skin barrier. That is a true genetic defect and it is very rare.

However, many children with inflammation in their skin are being subjected to genetic investigations which someone hopes will explain why the inflammation is happening. There seems to be a desire to justify the word *atopic* in eczema cases, especially in children. In a few cases a genuine genetic cause will be found. Yet I know one set of parents whose little boy was deemed to have a genetic defect and they were told it explained the duration and severity of his eczema. They were told to prepare themselves for him always having eczema. When they ended the boy's eczema, they were left wondering what all the genetic advice was about. They learned there was a perfectly good explanation for the inflammation without searching for elusive genetic changes to justify the atopic aspect. While his skin was out of balance, they were applying over a dozen products to his damaged skin. When they learned the significance of that, they stopped using those products, the eczema ended and his skin healed. He still has the same genes and now he has normal skin.

Diligently searching for complexity sometimes conceals simplicity. In this case there was no genetic defect to explain eczema; the patient was normal. Extremely refined genetic tests will reveal the variation within humans but does variation have to mean defect? No. It might simply show we're all different. Thank goodness for that! Yet those parents had been categorically told their child would always have eczema because of the genetic 'defect'. That distressed them at the time, although they laughed it off when their child's eczema disappeared inside two weeks and the alternative view of genetic tests was explained to them.

Inflammation in the skin

When eczema shows on the skin, it's generally assumed the inflammation is a result of the immune system 'going wrong' for some complicated and unexplainable reason. The word 'atopic' is used because those choosing to view eczema as a disease can't understand why the immune system is generating the inflammation. It's why drugs like steroids are used in eczema; to reduce what is seen as an unhelpful immune response. You now know there is another way of interpreting that skin inflammation.

With a different perspective, that inflammation can be seen as an excellent and perfectly appropriate response by the immune system as it tries to expel foreign material it has detected within the skin. Rather than the inflammation in eczema representing something 'wrong', try viewing it as an expected, desirable and totally appropriate response to chemical ingression and insult.

Using inflammation to expel foreign chemicals is part of the skin's healing process. In that regard, the inflammation in eczema is a good thing; it's the right response as the skin is doing its job of protecting the person against foreign chemicals which are in the wrong place.

There are ways of helping the skin perform that protection. Obviously if you avoid applying foreign chemicals, the skin won't have to protect the person from foreign chemicals which aren't there. That has been covered extensively already in this book.

Damaged skin can be cleansed with products which do *not* provoke the immune system when these products find their way down skin cracks. How do you tell which products do what? If you apply them and the skin is provoked into reacting with inflammation, those products provoke the immune system. That's easy. If you apply cleansing products to damaged skin and the inflammation goes away, those products do not provoke the immune system. Equally easy. Remember the statement that "if the skin doesn't like it the skin doesn't like it". Find something else the skin does like.

Within the skin are tiny blood vessels. The vessels coming to the skin bring oxygen and nutrients to the skin cells. Those going away from the skin carry away waste products.

There is another system of tiny vessels which help with the removal of waste products. These are the lymph vessels which begin in the skin and take waste to the lymph nodes for the body's version of forensic analysis. If a lymph node detects signs of something that should not be in the skin, it will induce more inflammation in the skin as part of the healing process.

The inflammation seen with eczema is a good thing as it's part of the skin's attempt to heal itself. Why, you might ask, is so much effort put into decreasing that inflammation with drugs like steroids? Wouldn't it be better to investigate why the inflammation in the skin is needed? Your utilisation of the 3 clues allows you to answer those questions. You can now come to your own realisations.

Massage

Gentle massage is another way to help skin perform its many tasks. Massage can increase the blood flow to the skin meaning more oxygen and nutrients reach the skin cells. It can also help the lymph vessels remove unwanted material created by the inner layer of skin cells.

Gentle massage is also very pleasurable. The nice effect goes deep, throughout the whole person. Sensations from the skin go to the brain which causes the release of special 'pleasure' compounds which induce bodily reactions varying from relaxation to excitement, depending on the situation. When parents massage their infants, one of the really beneficial results is an increase in the bond between the parent and child.

That is very good. What is not so good is the use of massage lubricants which go IN the skin and provoke the child's immune system into inflammation. Even though the parental massaging of the child was done with the best intentions, it is not good if the massage lubricant leads to eczema. The vast majority of the very well known and globally available products sold as skin lubricants contain high levels of chemical which is foreign to the human body. The most important point is the level of chemical content. When those chemicals remain ON the skin they simply make slippery skin. When they go IN the skin they can make eczema. Sadly, the extremely tiny skin cracks which precede dry skin are invisible; a parent can't see them. When those cracks are there, the massage lubricants which provoke the immune system become unfit for use.

In that situation, massage can lead to harm and very few parents want to harm their children.

The good news is that there are now massage lubricants which do not provoke the immune system to induce inflammation in the skin. It would be inappropriate to name them here as this book is available in many countries and those products may not be available in all the countries. However, using the knowledge in this book should allow people to determine which products are suitable.

Skin rashes

One of the most common skin rashes in children is simple heat rash. It may occur because the ambient room temperature is too high for the individual child. It may result from a very local warming in the flexure of the elbow or knee. It could occur around the edge of nappies/diapers where the garment prevents normal heat loss.

When a nappy/diaper rash occurs, it's often hard to decide whether the cause lies in the nappy touching the skin, heat not being able to leave the skin because of the nappy, bodily fluids soaking the skin or perhaps something like powder or other product that has been applied.

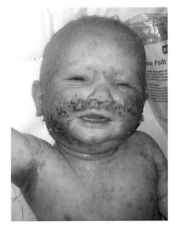

From the eczema perspective, it matters little how the skin rash arose. Once it's there, most products which are commonly applied to skin rashes in babies have the ability to provoke the immune system into inflammation against the products. Eczema then confuses the issue and the underlying cause of the first rash can be very hard to determine.

The child in this photograph has terrible eczema, especially on the face. As usual, that was very confusing.

However, have a close look at the redness in the armpit. That redness in the armpits was intermittent and could change within a day. That allowed us to realise the underlying issue for this boy's skin was actually the home being kept too warm for him. It was completely logical for the parents to want to keep a child with such skin ailments nice and warm, but it transpired that it was too warm for him. The redness in the armpits was a heat rash. When the temperature was lowered to match his preference, the heat rashes disappeared and the eczema ended soon after.

A similar sequence can occur with nappy/diaper rash, regardless of how the rash actually arises. Once the patch of skin is inflamed, it will be warmer making it more susceptible to heat from the surroundings. Applying many products to that hotter damaged area of skin runs the real risk of inducing eczema. In contrast, when such rashes are cleansed with water-based products which do not induce inflammation, the skin can heal itself.

Environmental chemicals

What other chemical factors from the outside might cause skin inflammation which can become the prelude to eczema? There are many; too many to list here. However you can use your imagination and experience to think of all the foreign chemicals that come into contact with skin.

A very limited list is:

- chemicals used to wash fabrics which contact the skin; clothes and bedclothes
- skin washes that are too aggressive for sensitive skin or are not properly washed off the skin
- shampoos which drain from the head downwards onto the rest of the skin
- environmental pollutants of many kinds which come into contact with the skin

- allergens the individual person reacts to
- household chemical products like washing-up-liquid and strong cleaning products.

You know how many more types of chemicals could be added to that list so I'll leave it there. The key point is that if those chemicals stay ON the skin and the immune system does not detect them, there will be no reason for inflammation. However when they go IN the skin and the immune system reacts to them, there will be inflammation. That early inflammation may have been a temporary malaise, but if products are applied to *manage* the inflammation you may turn a temporary skin rash into chronic eczema.

Food and drink

This is a good time to wonder what could affect skin from the inside. How do products reach the skin from within? Via the blood which flows to the skin. How do products get into the blood? One way is via what we swallow. Things we swallow rarely stay as they were prior to ingestion. What you swallow is usually broken down into smaller parts by digestion and the smaller parts are then absorbed from the intestines and taken by the blood to the liver for processing. Sometimes what we take in is fine but it's changed within the body into something which is problematic. An awful lot is going on within this context and very little of it need concern us here unless it affects the skin.

In relation to skin rashes and eczema, allow the skin to be the judge. If the skin does not react with inflammation when the person eats or drinks, that's fine. If you do get skin inflammation as a result of something which has been swallowed, then we have something to discuss. Sadly, when you enter into that discussion you enter the realms of massive complications. For example, how do patch tests performed on skin actually relate to the allergen when it's taken in by mouth and digested into its parts? There is an answer but it's seriously complicated. I read immunology journals where this is being discussed and have to admit that I come away dazed. Better informed, but definitely dazed.

Skin patch tests certainly have a role to play. What I want to point out here is how much confusion they can cause for parents.

The list of possible food allergens is as diverse as the people who react to them. Is there another way of addressing the association between food, drinks, allergies and eczema? Yes, there is.

This chapter is all about the holistic approach where the whole person is the subject. That's much more than just the skin, much more than any one organ. In a similar fashion, diet is much more than one nutrient. If you want to stay as close to a natural balance as you can, eat foods which are still as nature made them. Even that simple advice can have complications, with peanuts being a good example. They are natural, wholesome, unprocessed food. So far, so good. For people with an intense allergy to peanuts, they are lethal. Not so good.

For non-lethal foods, let the skin be the judge of whether a food is good for any individual person. Adverse reactions to cow milk, wheat, various fruits, soya and many other natural foods show why it's so unwise to dilute the key message in this book with masses of confusing debate over foods. If swallowing a particular food or drink induces inflammation in the skin, avoid that food or drink. It sounds simple, but rest assured I know how incredibly complicated that can be. But avoiding that simple message could lead to the massive complications of eczema.

If inflammation of the skin results from swallowing particular materials, don't swallow them. There are ample other foods to sustain a human. Simplifying to that extent may seem cruel to someone who craves a particular processed food, but when I'm being asked for advice on eczema I often find it necessary to convey such bad news.

To provide some balance, I like to say "everything should be taken in moderation, *especially* moderation".

The fact that one in five of our babies is diagnosed with eczema in their first 12 months of life is a frightening statistic. Something is clearly out of balance. Many of those babies will have been breast-fed so what they swallow has come from their mother. Any adverse reactions they have to breast milk will be a reaction to what the mother has consumed. I recall a first-time mother who diligently avoided her favourite hot curries during pregnancy and for many months while she was breast-feeding. When she did have a "fire-eating" curry she laughs about how 'characterful' the nappies were within hours. When her baby's skin turned red she found it less amusing. The really sad thing was how she then avoided all types of curry until the baby was fully weaned. That's sad because the baby had reacted to the REALLY hot curry whereas the mother could have enjoyed more normal curries, possibly to the benefit of the child. It is incredibly easy to make a balanced and very tasty home-made curry so the mother could have enjoyed her favourite food and the baby would have been exposed to a wider range of foods, all in balance.

In due course I plan to write a lot more about the relationship between eczema and what is swallowed. Until then, utilise the well trusted advice of enjoying a balanced diet;

- seek products high in omega 3 oils
- ensure you have some omega 6 oil as it is essential to health but keep it low as any excess is metabolised into pro-inflammatory compounds
- be aware that products with high glycemic indexes induce rapid and unhelpful rises in blood sugars and direct your preferences to more complex carbohydrates which are digested more slowly
- obtain a regular supply of easily digested proteins.

One useful clue is that an overdose of anything is an overdose, regardless of whether the specific thing is organic, natural, cooked or raw. The intention is a good balance and it's hard to balance when one component pushes others out of place.

A person should be able to enjoy what they eat and drink. Such joy is a fantastic way to deliver health and happiness. A healthy happy person who is in balance with their diet is more likely to be in balance with their skin. It's worth remembering the old saying that "eczema is what the person does rather than what they have". That is particularly relevant to what they swallow.

It's a sad fact that many people have not been taught to cook in a meaningful way. That can leave them dependent on processed foods which sometimes lead to inflammation of the skin. In many countries there are numerous celebrity chefs on television, most of whom show how easy it is to cook well from basic ingredients. Ironically it is now the high number of chefs that adds to the confusion. I like to direct people who want to learn how easy it is to cook well to Dale Pinnock. I enjoy using his book "The Medicinal Chef" as the recipes are really simple and easy to follow. If you can't find his book, go to his website www.dalepinnock.co.uk for recipes. People I direct to Dale tend to share very favourable comments on how he improves their lives.

Obviously there are other very helpful sources of advice on food. In due course I will be providing suggestions for people who opt for vegetarian and vegan eating styles. The important point in this section is that what people swallow can affect their skin. Yet it is only one of many factors and is best kept in perspective.

Stress

It is wisest to avoid offering any definition of stress. Those affected by it know what they believe it is and a very good way of increasing their stress is to provide them with another person's definition. Therefore, no definitions. I once knew a group conducting research into the body's reaction to stress. They banned the use of the word 'stress' in their laboratory as the word meant different things to different people. In order to make progress, they forced themselves to say exactly what they meant each time they were tempted to use the word. Nobody in that group was allowed to take the lazy option of using such an ambiguous confusing word.

But we need to accept it exists and the effect of stress can be patches of reddened skin, a rash.

The big question is what happens next? Does the debate swing towards what induced the skin redness in the belief that a good answer will allow you to end the rash? Or is the automatic reaction to apply skincare products onto the reddened area? The latter has become the norm; we have an entire industry suggesting that is a good habit to maintain. Once it happens, the cause of the redness is often obscured or not even investigated. If the products applied to the redness turn it into eczema, the discussion then centres on the inflammation and all its connotations. That is a terrible shame as there would have been some very useful clues to be found in the debate on why the rash appeared.

This is a good point to mention that the body responds to stress by producing steroids. These are essential chemicals in a balanced human and we make them at varying levels every day. They are basically the same steroids people like to hate in skincare products. It has been proven by medical research that a good bout of stress causes a measurable defect in the skin barrier. This happens because the inherent natural steroids reduce the ability of skin cells to make certain components necessary to form the skin barrier. As you know so well, defective skin barrier means chemicals can gain access to the skin leading to eczema. This explains why people often have a flare-up of eczema after being stressed.

Atopic March

It's widely accepted that eczema, asthma and hay fever are related. They are grouped as 'atopic' diseases since some people find it hard to explain why the immune system is reacting the way it is. A person who has any of the three is said to be 'atopic'. It's reported that if both parents are atopic, there is a 90% chance their child will develop eczema. That implies a genetic link which is now often reinforced by genetic tests on the child.

Atopic people with only one or two of the atopic conditions often despair of being told they will develop the ones they don't yet have. It is an assumption; something they can't do anything about. It is a way of thinking.

Yet I suggest the inflammation in eczema is NOT atopic. It can be explained quite easily in most cases. Let's look at that another way because my view is proving to be a tremendous challenge to many of those who manage eczema. I suggest the inflammation is due to foreign chemicals which have found their way IN the skin where the immune system detects them and reacts with inflammation. If anyone wants to challenge that logic, I like to ask if they believe those foreign chemicals could reside in the skin *without* any response from the immune system? None of the challengers has said yes.

It is also worth pointing out that some people who used to have the full set of three atopic diseases; eczema, asthma and hay fever, no longer have eczema. They are now EXeczema successes yet they still have asthma and hay fever. I feel that reinforces my view that eczema is not 'atopic'. It is an expected immune reaction to foreign chemicals gaining access to the skin. It's most likely those products were actively and deliberately applied. The effect we see when those chemicals provoke the immune system into reacting with inflammation is easily explained. In fact it is a desirable process intended to defend the patient.

Being a romantic, I like to believe there are individuals like me somewhere in the world providing the same hope for asthma and hay fever. It would be wonderful if simple answers to prevent asthma and hay fever were presented, wouldn't it? I suggest optimism.

Anti-scratch psychology

An extremely persistent itch is part of eczema. That presents the risk of the patient scratching through their skin leading to broken skin and bleeding. In a few individuals, even when the redness due to Product Maintained Dermatitis is gone, the overall itch can continue.

The medical term for itch is Pruritis and so far the drug companies have yet to offer a drug solution. Antihistamines are commonly prescribed even though they are not directly intended to work against this problem. Histamine is a natural compound produced in inflammation so antihistamines are simply aiming to reduce one small part of the overall inflammation. We have discussed how the inflammation itself is only one part of the eczema cycle. However, when people lack the wherewithal to address the full cycle, there can be advantage in them working to reduce small individual components in the hope of affecting the whole imbalance. That is the reason steroids are used to reduce the inflammation. It is the same when antihistamines are prescribed to reduce one aspect of one component. The logic goes that at least it's something and if you lack a better understanding of what's actually going on then it's best to do something.

It is now widely recognised that the antihistamines which cause drowsiness aid the itch problem by helping children achieve deeper, more prolonged, sleep. In effect, those antihistamines are used as sedatives. That achieves a purpose in reducing the damage caused by unconscious scratching at night. It also serves a purpose in showing how far the drug industry is from providing a directed answer for the intense itch in eczema.

A tool that can work if it's provided by suitably skilled personnel is psycho-therapy to teach the patient how to resist the desire to scratch their itch. In terms of simple psychology, just instructing someone to "stop scratching" usually results in them scratching even more. One step up from that is coaching to let them know they are welcome to scratch, and then anchor the negative effect of scratching with the sensation of itch. Done well, this allows the patient to associate itch with pain and in due course the thought of pain reduces the natural impulse to scratch an itch.

The psycho-therapy I am referring to here is several layers above this. I am deliberately not providing many details for several reasons:

1. Each professional psycho-therapist has their own way of guiding a patient and if I preempt their steps here I can hamper their chances of achieving success.
2. If a therapist can provide relief from the itch and that reduces the self-trauma from scratching, it's best to let them do it.
3. The itch is the result of the inflammation which in most cases is the result of foreign chemicals IN the skin. The body's natural defence strategy is to use inflammation against those chemicals and one part of the inflammation is itch. The real question is why the chemicals are in such an inappropriate place? Working on the itch alone means those managing the person's overall imbalance have yet to address the fundamental issue.

Psycho-therapy to reduce the desire to scratch the itch in eczema is a really useful and successful tool. It was very appropriate when atopic eczema could justifiably be called atopic. Having progressed this far through the book, you may now question whether the inflammation in atopic eczema is unexplainable or in the wrong place? If you believe the inflammation can be explained as a natural and perfectly proper immune response to foreign chemicals being in the wrong place IN the skin, you no longer favour the use of the word atopic with eczema. Your new knowledge has allowed you to progress and view the imbalance with a completely different perspective. You may find it more beneficial to prevent the cause of the skin inflammation rather than manage one small part of one symptom of the imbalance.

Or you may prefer to find a psycho-therapist who can break the itch-scratch cycle while you leave the underlying cause as it is and manage the eczema.

Choice

As you know so well by now, I like using psychology to provide people with choices. Part of that lies in letting them realise what choices they have available, and especially helping them find the ones that are new to them. Those new choices will have probably always been there but until they become apparent they are unavailable to the person.

Atopic eczema is now a disease of choice; manage it or end it. Some manage it; most end it. That raises the choice of positioning yourself in the larger group containing individual successes or the smaller group with no successes. It's a choice. Prior to reading this book you may not have been aware this choice was available to you. Now you know it is.

Saying atopic eczema is a disease of choice raises all sorts of reactions varying from relief to condemnation. I find the condemnation most interesting when it comes from those who have chosen to avoid investigating my work and learn why I am saying what I say. They have chosen to resist gaining some new knowledge which is freely available. As you can imagine, among that group are people who dislike me associating the word *manage* with *maintain* in relation to eczema. That is their choice and I like people to have choices.

When doctors' choices adversely affect patients with eczema, they find themselves in a whole new debate on medical ethics. If they deliberately take actions which keep a person in a state of imbalance leading to a sustained medical condition like eczema, it's a choice they have taken. The alternative choice to end that person's eczema may not have been apparent to them before. This book means it is now. That raises new choices for them. They can choose to argue with my thesis, suggest improvements to overcome weaknesses in my argument or encompass the ideas. This book offers them new choices.

If their choice brings them into conflict with medical ethics I take the choice to back away. As you will have seen from my degrees, I am not a medical doctor. I am a PhD, a philosopher, a thinker. I gain a lot of my new knowledge by conversing with people and asking questions. Their answers provide me with many choices which I then share with others.

One choice was for me to write this book and the fact that you're reading it indicates success.

I asked people who had ended their eczema what they had done just prior to the skin redness going away. Their diverse answers provided clues on how the skin imbalance had been ended. In time I used that information to realise how the eczema began. That new discovery provided, as you might expect, another choice. In view of how challenging my new realisation would be for those who believe eczema is atopic and incurable, I could remain quiet or set out to help explain eczema. You know my choice was to help.

EXeczema® Success

Bethan's hard-won happiness

"Have you been swimming?" This was the question frequently asked by people on seeing Bethan with her greasy, limp hair caused by the use of thick emollients.

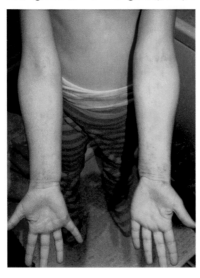

It was starting school that really saw a decline in Bethan's skin. After seeing a Consultant Dermatologist our life became one huge routine of creaming, wet-wrapping, ticking encouragement charts, packing a large box of treatments every time we went away, wearing 'magic pyjamas', writing action plans for the school and educating family members. Watching Bethan withdraw into herself with such low self esteem made me realise we were desperate and ready to try anything.

We have tried alternative ways to treat it; homeopathy, aloe vera plants, salt baths, oat baths etc. Life turned a corner when we met a revolutionary and inspirational doctor at the Norfolk eczema support group. He introduced us to his EXeczema theory. With my professional knowledge of physiology and the chance to speak one to one with Dr Harley, the theory made so much sense. Understanding how the skin works and heals itself was enlightening. With his support we radically changed the management of Bethan's skin.

At the time this process was difficult. The programme was in the infant stages and we were very willing 'guinea pigs'. The first two weeks went to plan, then the 'itch' came and nearly stopped us in our tracks. However, Bethan aged 7 refused to turn back to those creams and I was determined or stubborn to see it through as I understood the potential.

Thank goodness we did. It took about 6 months to say we were out of eczema. No products, no nagging to stop scratching, it feels as if a huge psychological weight has been lifted. Bethan's withdrawn nature nearly immediately reversed and confidence in herself rose . Interestingly, I also joined in on the programme, stopped all body lotions and use the NewGenn handwash. For the first time in years, my 'normal dry skin' does not flake during winter.

Two and a half years on we still use the handwash and wipes as a family and there is no mention of eczema anymore.

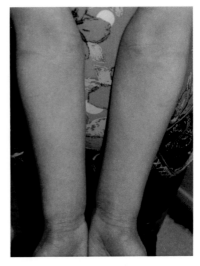

Bethan's notes: I'm so glad my eczema has gone now (all thanks to Dr Harley and my family's support). I am now more popular at school, and the horrible bullying and teasing has stopped. My hair is now long, wavy and a lighter colour than before.

Clothes are now not blood-covered and greasy (due to the creams).

And, if it hadn't been for Dr Harley, I would be still performing the routine of mum and dad creaming me daily, and greasy, wet-looking hair. I feel more confident, happier and pleased my eczema has gone.

Kath and Bethan 2014

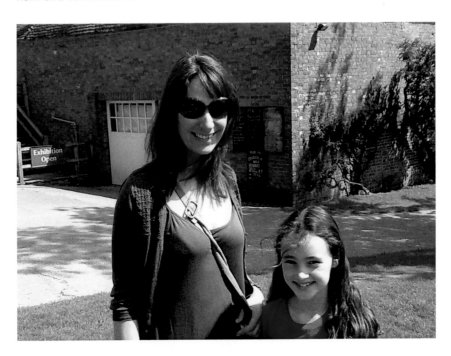

CHAPTER 11

Thoughts count

You are now very close to the end of this book. You have found a way through the many boundaries I deliberately laid on your path! A bit sneaky of me really so I'll beg a tiny bit of forgiveness. The intention was to challenge you while simultaneously ensuring you could visualise the goal of EXeczema. The time after eczema is a new concept to many sufferers and seeing people reach it is a wonderful feeling. Looking into the eyes of a child who has just been released from the incessant misery of eczema generates a wonderful feeling inside.

That feeling, and the ability to share it by having others free more children, is what fuels the global EXeczema® campaign. It has already reached the point where I personally don't get to know most of the success cases. There is great excitement in the way the campaign is spreading around the world encouraging others to join, spreading health and happiness.

You have now reached the end of this happy story. If you want to read the challenges I'm posing to the established treatment paradigms, you will see them in the final chapter. You can enjoy the happy ending and help others reach their new goal without reading and knowing those challenges. Equally, you may find it helps your resolve to know how the most up to date science I've incorporated into the campaign is helping so many people move forward. As you might expect, and I always hope, there will be some in every group who challenge my challenges. That generates discussion. It encourages new questions and I love new questions as they're a fantastic way of revealing new answers. Avoiding the discussions leaves us without questions and then we prevent ourselves from having the answers. If there was no eczema remaining around the world it wouldn't really matter if we ignored the discussions, questions and answers. But there is still a huge problem to be overcome, isn't there?

The medical library where I do most of my investigative research has a journal room the size of a tennis court with row after row of journals with each row being two metres high. There is an enormous amount of information for those who seek it. In recent times more and more journals are only being published on-line which simply means you access them via a computer. The amount of information continues to grow at an exponential rate making it an ever greater challenge to find the single gem of an idea you want. Despite that, the opportunity to find your gem is still there.

Saying information is "on the internet" has somehow belittled the magnitude of what's available. The internet certainly makes it easier to search for the things others are searching for. That's how search-engines work; they hone in on the more commonly asked questions. However, finding the gem that others haven't thought of seeking means you need to utilise your own investigative efforts. After all, if "eczema can't be cured" how much funding do you think is made available to researchers with an idea on how to cure eczema? Very little. Funding for research has always worked in a similar fashion to the way search-engines work now. Just as search-engines reflect the trends of what people are asking at the time, research funding has always followed trends of what's being asked in the specific sphere of interest.

If the question you are interested in is not a prominent part of the wider discussion, it would be naive to hope the answer would be obvious in the journals. The skill lies in generating a very specific question. When you're presuming the answer you need is waiting to be found, each little failure provides the clues to success. If you can't find the answer or if you don't find the answer useful, the skill lies in re-visiting the question. One of the best ways is to divide the question into smaller parts. Eventually you will have a series of exceedingly specific questions and answers to go with them. Then you use the answers as you would bricks when you're building a wall. The bricks you find this way will almost certainly be of many different sizes and you need to develop the skill of making something strong and useful from such diverse shapes.

Most walls are made of conventional highly uniform bricks and therefore all look basically the same. Since that is what's usually required, that's ideal. However, when conventional is not serving people well, something different is needed. The materials to build a different looking wall are out there. They just need to be found, evaluated and then carefully put into a useful pattern. It can be done but very few allow the time to do it.

The EXeczema programme is very much like that different wall. Conventional bricks have been used for years and millions of eczema sufferers are trapped by the resultant conventional walls. Those walls represent the mental boundaries, and those boundaries are set by people other than the sufferers. The people who set the boundaries are saying "we know best and you can't escape." Obviously they are not using those precise words, but might the much repeated phrase "*you* can't cure eczema" amount to the same thing?

If that negative statement leads to limiting beliefs and mental boundaries which constrain eczema sufferers, then it acts as a wall. Since the same negative statement is being heard around the world, it becomes the convention. It morphs into best medical practice. It becomes established. Many come to see it as fact and the negative is proven.

Yet, as any good researcher knows, you can't prove a negative. People setting out on a research career are taught to use what we call a null hypothesis. Since you can't prove a negative like "you can't cure eczema" the correct path is to form the null hypothesis of "you can cure eczema" and work to prove it wrong.

This may seem needlessly complicated but please trust me for a little longer.

Many millions of people are constrained by the negative statement that you can't cure eczema. They are told to just accept it because all the research supports the negative with the presumption that the negative has been proven.

Yet they should know they can't prove a negative. Do you find that interesting? So many influential people are stating what the rest of us are supposed to believe is fact. Yet they haven't proven it.

If they can't prove the negative statement that you can't cure eczema, it's not a fact at all. There can be no research to prove it. So what is all that research about? If I know they haven't even utilised the most fundamental tool of good research, a valid null hypothesis, why do I spend so much time looking through so many articles and journals?

Because the answer to the wrong question is still an answer. Remember, I have a deeply held conviction that the answers I want are out there. All I need do is find the right questions. To me it doesn't matter how relevant to my interests their question was or how valid their answers are if they haven't used a valid null hypothesis. The useful bit lies in the fact that they publish their answers. When I create a new question, I go trawling through their answers to find any that fit my newest question. Often the answers don't quite fit as well as needed, so I re-visit my most recent question. I usually sub-divide it into more specific questions. Then I find answers for those.

If you're thinking this might be incredibly time consuming, then *please congratulate yourself!* You are absolutely correct. It takes ages. For the EXeczema programme, it took several years.

Why do I feel this is relevant for readers of this book? Because one of the thoughts which blocks many people is why the researchers and eczema advisers didn't find the answers which form the basis of the positive story. Do you recall a little question earlier in the book which went something like "If it's so simple, why haven't others found it before?" Have you met many eczema advisers with plenty of spare time? I certainly haven't. If you know some researchers, do you know any with spare time? Again, I don't. In fact they all tend to be incredibly busy generating results which conform to the conventional trend on which their next funding will be based.

I have the privilege of time. I've spent my career creating time for this type of endeavour. Now I have my own company where my main role is to find time and use it to good effect doing this. Creating the EXeczema campaign has required a huge amount of time; a resource most others lack for many valid reasons. That's why the conventional teams have failed to find the simple answers. They were charged with finding a complicated answer to a complicated problem. It's therefore hardly surprising they didn't see a simple answer to a simple problem. The answer was always there; the right question was eluding them.

The final chapter is something I want the relevant people around the world to read and discuss. It is less important to those who like this story and the happy ending, those who are keen to spread the "we did" story. The last chapter is written in the hope that influencers in the medical world will challenge my ideas. If they find sufficient errors in my logic to destroy my thesis, I will use their comments to begin again. However, if they can't prove me wrong, I invite them to wonder if I'm right. If I am right, then my challenges to their treatment paradigms warrant action. A lack of action at that point will be very significant. Continuing to support paradigms which are not in the best interests of their patients means a lot. If those paradigms are actually harming patients, that means a lot more. That would lead into troubled waters, to put it politely.

It pays to listen. It's also polite and beneficial to both the speaker and the listener. The speaker can have a lot to say. The listener can learn a lot.

It also pays to question, as long as you really listen to the answer. You may find that having given due consideration to the answer, you find yourself with a new question. To people like me who value philosophy and diverse thinking, this never-ending supply of new questions is exciting. I'm very lucky in being able to make time for new questions and the answers they deliver. I appreciate how few share that privilege.

The dominant view of those who advise on eczema is that "eczema can't be cured." As you know I ask if they are really saying "**we** can't" cure eczema? If they can't, they are allowed to ask who can. If they don't ask they are unlikely to find the answer. It is a skill which needs to be developed and one which takes a lot of time.

Now consider that huge group of people, including me, who ended their eczema long ago and thereafter kept it in remission and had healthy skin. That suits my definition of cure. I have cured my eczema. As have millions and millions of others around the world in recent decades. In effect we are saying "we did" cure eczema.

Compare those two statements: "we can't" and "we did". Both are correct. Those who can't, can't. Those who did, did.

Would you expect a positive outcome to arise from what's being discussed in the "we can't" or the "we did" group? Remember both groups are correct. Both are doing the best they can with the resources they have available. One such resource is choice and this book serves to provide the "we can't" group with new choices. If they opt to ignore the new choices, that is a choice in itself.

This book means eczema is now a matter of choice; *manage* it or *end* it.

Whether a product is ON the skin or IN the skin makes a huge difference. Nobody has ever proven that statement wrong. At the moment, that's my main contribution to the global eczema debate. The rest of this book stems from that one statement.

When the next skin rash appears, as it will for everyone, those with the knowledge gained here will know how to prevent the skin rash turning into eczema. Even if they try a product which sadly does cause eczema, they know how to end that eczema because they've succeeded before and they can succeed again.

The sheer simplicity of my statement regarding ON or IN raises questions. Those who value new questions are delighted to find new and useful answers. They earn themselves the choice of using their new answers. Those who prefer to ignore new questions prevent themselves from gaining the choice to use the new answers.

Speaking to you as someone who knows a lot about skin, please allow me to end with a question.

Whether a product is **ON** the skin or **IN** the skin makes a huge difference, doesn't it?

EXeczema® Success

Daniel Sutcliffe takes control

I started with eczema in 2008 at the age of 26, with a red rash around my eyes. Over the next few years, I was prescribed various and ever-stronger steroids and countless creams and lotions. But my condition became worse, eventually spreading over my entire body. By the end of 2012 I was stuck – the steroids and moisturisers no longer had any short term improving effects. That's when I came across EXeczema. Suddenly it all made sense. The very medication I'd been prescribed to try and 'control' this condition were actually perpetuating it and making it worse.

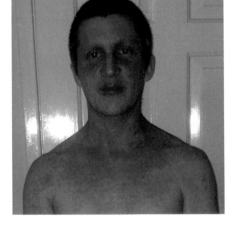

Within 48 hours of ceasing all topical treatments, I was a big red flaky mess. Gradually, over 3 or 4 months, this improved. After 4 months my skin was able to tolerate a family holiday to Portugal, and the sunshine and sea helped me improve further. I remember my wife commenting at the time, "I've got my husband back".

Unfortunately after around 9 months I had a big set-back, with oozing skin returning on my face and other areas. I think this was partly stress related, as both my children were quite poorly and so I spent a lot of time in hospitals. I managed to pick up a persistent infection that took 7 weeks of antibiotics to clear.

It is now about 20 months since I took control of my skin and stopped listening to the medical establishment. I am so glad that I did. I sometimes wonder what a mess I would be in if I had continued using damaging steroids and continued to bombard my immune system with creams and lotions. The journey I have been

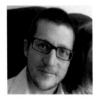

on has been the hardest thing I have ever done, but I also know it's one of the best things I've ever done in terms of my own health.

I still have a few issues – hands, feet and the backs of knees. I still have a scratching problem with my hands and feet. But these areas are still improving month by month. I also get the occasional bit of dry skin on my face, scalp and lips, but really this is pretty minor.

P.S. I thought you might like to include the sentences in one of my recent emails to you.

"It is now just over 2 years since I first contacted you. Back then I couldn't image what today would be like".

CHAPTER 12

Questions on paradigms

This chapter is written predominantly for those providing advice on eczema, although its inclusion here makes it readily available to all readers. It summarises what has been presented already and therefore you will find repetition. That is deliberate and done because I have found it useful in the many coaching exercises I've undertaken while developing the EXeczema® programme.

Eczema is a very common condition which has been prominent for many years. Patient care has evolved into set paradigms covering best practices supported by evidence-based research. If that patient care has resulted in treatment regimes which *maintain* the disease, does it become relevant to ask whether the 'evidence' is evidence of *success* or evidence of *failure*?

That question is provided in the interests of encouraging debate. Those who choose to reject it out of hand will know why the've taken that action. Only they can know their reasons as they've excluded themselves from this debate. Those who agree with the question or challenge in a constructive manner will improve the thesis leading, I believe, to a great reduction in the number of eczema sufferers.

My challenges to the paradigms will mean very little to anyone who has not read the main body of this book. Anyone who opts to challenge my thoughts without knowing the basis of the thinking will negate their contribution to the debate. That really will be sad as we would all benefit from informed inclusion.

What paradigms do I believe warrant challenge?

1. Most eczema is atopic.
2. Opaque emollients help the patient.
3. Hydrophobic moisturisers help the patient.
4. Topical steroids are to the long-term benefit of eczema patients.

5. It helps to reinforce the atopic march.
6. Eczema patients will have a genetic defect if you search hard enough.

Most eczema is atopic.

Atopic eczema is the name given to the most common form of eczema as it's believed there's no justifiable explanation for the inflammation. I came to question that choice of name when parents told me I had 'cured' eczema in their children. Whatever effect I'd had was unintentional. While working in the field of infection prevention in hospitals, I led a team that created a range of antibacterial skincare products which left a very pleasant feeling on skin. The intention was to generate a positive feedback loop every time the products were used in order to encourage better user compliance. Without me being aware of it, those products were used to cleanse the skin of children with eczema. Within weeks, the eczema had disappeared.

That *anecdotal* evidence induced me to compare the ingredients in our products with those in products which had been used while the eczema was present. Our products contained an absolute minimum of chemical content as I wanted them to be mostly water. Most of the other products contained high levels of chemicals, especially mineral oils which I knew induced intense inflammation when detected by the immune system. It has been shown that when they permeate the skin barrier they disrupt the lipid bilayers essential to skin barrier function.

If I could find a way for the immune system to detect the provocative ingredients in those topical skincare products, I would have found a justification for the inflammation in eczema.

In fact it was easy.

i. Eczema presents as patches of damaged skin. There is increased TEWL (TransEpidermal Water Loss) in eczema-affected skin. That is explained by the capacity of the skin barrier being suboptimal so more water is lost from eczema-affected skin than from adjacent areas of non-inflamed skin. The affected areas of skin are deemed to be more porous. If more water than usual is getting out, foreign chemicals are more able to get in.

ii.   Eczema tends to follow and be associated with xerosis, dryness of skin. Prior to xerosis being perceived by the patient, there will be tiny cracks in the *stratum corneum*, the outermost layer of the epidermis. Those skin cracks reduce the skin's physical barrier to chemical ingression. Chemicals applied to areas of xerosis will be able to enter the cracks. If the cracks are deep enough for the foreign chemicals to be detected by the immune system, there will be inflammation. That is the expected and desired response to foreign material in the skin.

Therefore, an eczema sufferer will have areas of skin with epidermal cracks making those areas more permeable than normal. That will allow ingredients in topical skincare products to enter the skin where the immune system can be relied upon to perform its intended function and react with inflammation.

In that regard, can the inflammation in eczematous patches of skin be explained? I believe it can. If this explanation of the inflammation makes sense to you, would you agree that it becomes wise to challenge the paradigm that *atopic* eczema is actually inflammation in the wrong place and hard to explain: atopic?

Opaque emollients are the best for patients.

Patients with eczema are advised to apply emollients to their skin regularly, even when their eczema is in remission and their skin looks normal. The current paradigm is that emollients help the patient so doctors and others advising people on how to manage eczema recommend emollients. The commonly used emollients are therefore associated with ongoing eczema; managing eczema.

What if those emollients are part of the problem? What if the immune system reacts to them with inflammation? Might those emollients be maintaining eczema?

There is rarely any constructive value in naming ingredients within a topic like this. Yet there is value in finding a way to differentiate between emollients which seem to provoke inflammation and those which don't. The simplest way I've found is to distinguish between opaque emollients, those you can't see through, and clear emollients which are transparent. Opacity versus clarity.

By definition of the word emollient, both opaque and clear versions moisturise the skin.

Opaque emollients have a high content of chemicals foreign to the human body providing more opportunity for them to provoke the immune system into inflammation. In contrast, the clear emollients available at the time of writing this book contain *very* low levels of chemicals. The fact that skin inflammation disappears with the use of these clear emollients would appear to be in the interests of patients. That suggests an advantage of clarity over opacity from the patient perspective.

There are very few clear, transparent, emollients available for advisors to recommend at the moment. However, they do exist. One of the reasons why I prefer to not name them lies in the fact that some clear emollients actually contain a HIGH level of chemical content. The key message here lies in the knowledge which allows people to let skin be the judge.

If the skin "doesn't like a product the skin doesn't like it". This is well known in the field of managing eczema as patients are advised to cease using an emollient to which the skin reacts. They are told to try another one. Sadly patients go from one emollient to another in a desperate search for one which does not induce inflammation in eczematous patches. By definition that suggests the emollients they have been using are maintaining the inflammation. By another definition if they happened to find an emollient which did not induce inflammation their eczema would have ended.

Given that opaque emollients are associated with prolongation of the inflammation and clear emollients are associated with the inflammation ending, would it be wise to advance from opacity to clarity? Advisors could still recommend the frequent and regular use of emollients but the very low level of chemical content in the clear versions means there is very little to provoke the immune system.

Now that there is a choice between opaque emollients with high chemical levels and clear emollients with very low chemical levels, would you agree it's valid to question the paradigm that opaque emollients are the best for patients?

Hydrophobic moisturisers help eczema patients.

To introduce this paradigm, I would like you to consider severe eczema on the back of a child's knee. In order for this exercise to work best, visualise that area of eczematous skin as being damaged, inflamed and wet to the point of oozing. The current treatment paradigm is that this damaged patch of skin must be kept moist and scabs should be avoided. That makes moisturisers a valid part of any attempt to manage eczema. That is the current paradigm for a patch of eczema on the back of that child's knee.

Now relocate your thoughts to the front of the same knee after the child has grazed its knee. There will be a patch of skin that is damaged, inflamed and wet to the point of oozing. Yet we like to let that area of damaged skin dry out. We know that once it's dry, scabs will form and those scabs are a beneficial part of the skin's healing process. As we know from life's experiences, when those scabs fall off, normal healthy skin will be revealed.

Why do we have such a difference in approach to wet damaged skin on the back of that knee and the front? The child's skin heals itself quickly when it's allowed to dry out and scab over. What's happening on the back of that knee to retard the inherent natural healing process?

What if the moisturisers were playing a part in prolonging the eczema? Is it possible that ingredients in those moisturisers are finding a way down cracks in the damaged skin leading to more inflammation with accompanying oozing? We know there is increased water loss in eczema patches as a result of the inflammation. What if the moisturisers were involved in causing that inflammation and subsequent increased water loss?

With that sequence in mind, is the moisturiser helping the patient? Or is the moisturiser maintaining the state of imbalance? To help I will approach the paradigm from another angle.

Traditional moisturisers are based on hydrophobic ingredients that repel water, a very common example being mineral oils. The logic suggests that when they are applied to the skin, they will reduce or even prevent the flow of water out through the skin; they repel the water, keeping it in the skin so trans-epidermal water flow will be reduced. But in eczema, when these water-repelling products are applied, there is an *increase* in trans-epidermal water loss. It seems a contradiction has arisen within this paradigm.

That contradiction is easily explained if the moisturisers are entering the skin, inducing inflammation which reduces the capacity of the skin barrier to hold water. Given that mineral oils are undeniably foreign to the human body, will they provoke inflammation if they penetrate the skin to the level where they're detected by the immune system? Yes.

Another consideration is the medical evidence that when hydrophobic mineral oils enter the skin they intercalate into, and disrupt the function of, the lipid bilayers in the skin barrier. That disruption will induce greater skin barrier permeability resulting in increased TEWL and enhanced entry of immunogenic medicament ingredients. The hydrophobic moisturisers induce the problem they were intended to reduce.

Is it time to challenge the paradigm that these hydrophobic moisturisers help eczema patients? Yes, but it would be immoral to just leave the patients with drying, itchy skin that invokes scratching which can create more skin damage. Therefore some more constructive thought is required to serve these patients well.

The logic of traditional moisturisers is that they contain hydrophobic chemicals which are supposed to hold water in the skin by preventing its evaporation. Is it conceivable that water can be added to the skin from the outside? Yes, of course it is. Might this offer a constructive way of keeping the skin moist? It could and it does; when products with a very high water content are used on the skin as moisturisers. Such an alternative choice now exists.

Would you agree this an opportunity to challenge this paradigm that hydrophobic moisturisers help eczema patients?

Topical steroids are to the long-term benefit of eczema patients.

For this part to be pertinent, please return to how we manage the eczema inflammation on the back of that child's knee and compare it to how we manage the graze on the front of the same knee. We do not attempt to reduce the inflammation on the front of the grazed knee even though it is damaged, inflamed, oozing skin. There was nothing wrong with the immune system on the front of the knee so we leave the immune system to protect the child. We allow the skin to heal itself.

Why do we use steroids to reduce inflammation on the back of the same knee when we know there is nothing wrong with the child's immune system? Is it because that area of damaged skin is called eczema? Is it because the prolonged heightened immune response is deemed to be acting against the child? Could it be there is no logical explanation for the inflammation on the back of the knee and therefore we're forced to call it 'atopic' and resort to active immuno-suppressing drugs like steroids? I'll leave you to provide answers to those questions if you want. Personally I see them as rhetorical questions once the logic in this book has been considered and assimilated.

We use immuno-suppressing steroids because that's what the current treatment paradigms suggest we must do, even when it can be easily argued that treating the immune response is so obviously just treating one symptom and avoiding the underlying cause of the inflammation.

There are perfectly good alternatives to steroids when immuno-suppression is essential. Calcineurin inhibitors are effective yet once again it is appropriate to ask whether the therapist should be focussing on just one of the symptoms.

When the eczema is severe, it's deemed appropriate to use cyclosporin to really dampen down the inflammation. That is a toxic drug and therefore can only be prescribed by specialists. When this is done, is it an attempt to treat the whole underlying condition or just a way of alleviating one aspect of a wider malaise? It is the latter.

We would not use such drugs to decrease the chances of inflammation expelling a splinter of wood from within the skin. Yet we use them in a way which reduces the chances of inflammation expelling foreign chemicals from within the skin. That distinction makes it appropriate to at least question this paradigm, wouldn't you agree?

There can be no doubt that intensive medical therapy is required for a child who is scratching severely eczematous skin to the point of allowing bacterial entry to the blood. Once septicaemia has occurred, the child's life must be saved with intensive use of antibiotic therapy. That will provide short-term benefits; it will be treating the consequence of the eczema rather than the eczema itself. Is reducing the inflammation doing the same? It is. Yes, there are times when it's essential to use strong immuno-suppressive drugs to save the patient's life, but are we forced to do that more frequently than we like because we've chosen to ignore that eczema is more than one or two of its component symptoms?

Even with mild eczema, we know using steroid creams does not end eczema; the steroid merely decreases the inflammation we now realise the cream can be causing. Why are we so content to pursue a course where we're likely to be causing the adverse changes we prefer to believe we're treating?

To challenge this important point, when the steroids are carried in vehicles made up of chemicals that are foreign to the human body, can those chemicals find their way down cracks in the damaged skin leading to inflammation against those chemicals? You know they can and we're gambling as to whether they will or not. Gambling in this context is an interesting choice in patient care.

An important additional consideration is the medical evidence which proves topical glucocorticoids decrease the capacity of keratinocytes to secrete ceramide lipids required for the formation of the skin barrier. This proves steroids are actively involved in reducing the capacity of the skin barrier which means steroids enhance the chances of immunogenic medicament ingredients entering the skin leading to product maintained dermatitis; eczema. Steroids have a role to play in reducing inflammation but it has to be accepted that they also play a role in the pathogenesis of eczema. Calcineurin inhibitors are available so we need to question why steroids are ever used in eczema given the published evidence of how they are involved in the pathogenesis of eczema.

Care-givers who prefer prevention over treatment will value the benefits in avoiding the inflammation. When that's done, there's no need to suppress the immune response as there won't be any inflammation to suppress. However, wouldn't you agree that treating the inflammation with products which can induce that inflammation is acting against the patient?

This is often dismissed as a circular argument in which the

patient occasionally spirals out of the mundane eczema cycle into potentially lethal septicaemia. That's melodramatic enough to close the debate for some people. It might also be the reason so many patients remain trapped in the eczema cycle, forever prone to spiralling into septicaemia. Those who see their role as forever waiting to dramatically treat the septicaemia may lose focus on the ability to simply prevent the whole process.

When treating a single symptom of the malady is the primary objective, decreasing the immune response for short-term gain seems reasonable. When ending the whole condition is the primary objective, the thinking moves several steps ahead of the inflammation and its cause. That is the choice; manage the eczema in such a way that inflammation in caused and needs to be reduced, or end the eczema so there is no inflammation.

That choice has existed for a long time. Would you agree it's time to challenge the paradigm that reducing the inflammation is to the long-term benefit of eczema patients?

It helps to reinforce the atopic march.

Eczema, asthma and hay fever are three diseases where the heightened immune response is deemed to be hard to comprehend. These are often called the three atopic diseases. A person who has one is considered more likely to develop the rest. That progression from one to three is the 'atopic march' which can become a self-fulfilling prophecy if patients resign themselves to it. Certainly people with eczema don't tend to be surprised when they also develop asthma or hay fever. They've been led to see it as inevitable; just what they knew would happen.

How then can we explain those patients who had all three of the atopic diseases, a full set of the 'atopic march', and then ended their eczema with the EXeczema® programme? They came to realise it was not necessary to have eczema. They came to appreciate a choice; to continue managing eczema as they were told they should, or end it as they came to realise they could.

I choose to avoid commenting on the role of the immune system in asthma and hay fever. There may still be an element of inevitability of one leading to the other. As a romantic, I like to believe there will be someone out there doing for asthma and hay fever what I'm doing for eczema; using a thorough understanding of the diseases to show they are needless and avoidable. For now I will simply say that romantic view is more realistic than many believe.

The only inevitable thing I see in the atopic march is that people who have all three conditions can end their eczema. They will continue to have sensitive skin and continue to be susceptible to certain products when they're applied to the skin. I know this from my personal experience. When I want to experiment on myself I use any one of many skincare products to cause a patch of eczema on myself. I deliberately cause Product Maintained Dermatitis. The reason I don't call that a flare-up of my eczema is that I'm completely in control of the sequence from deciding to cause it to deciding when to end it. I even control the level of severity I want. Sadly, patients trapped in the eczema cycle lack that control, *until* they learn what is happening in their skin.

Those who choose to study the technical scientific details in the Appendix will learn of a train of thought which suggests severe early-onset eczema can predispose a patient to developing asthma and hay fever. There is good evidence to support that sequence. However, should that happen in an individual patient, my suggestion is that the understanding and knowledge presented here will enable them still to end their eczema.

I therefore believe it is time to challenge the paradigm that its good for the patient to reinforce the atopic march; to instil a limiting belief that the full set of atopic conditions is somehow inevitable.

Eczema now comes with a choice. Plenty of people fulfil the atopic march expectation by having all three of the atopic march conditions. I hope many of them will come to realise at least one of the three is being maintained by the products they are using to manage it.

Eczema patients will have a genetic defect if you search hard enough

We are now blessed with some wonderful ways of examining a person's genetic code. Those genetic tests represent a true advance in science and medicine.

To me, the challenge arises in the way we choose to interpret results from these tests. A family I know was told a translocation on one of their son's chromosomes meant he would always have eczema. That change in his chromosome was the justification for the duration of his chronic skin disease. When they ended their son's eczema within two weeks, an interesting situation arose. There was obviously no change in the boy's genetic makeup and he would still have his translocation, yet his eczema was gone and he has stayed in remission for years. He has had skin rashes since and his parents use their new knowledge to keep them as skin rashes, all of which disappeared. He still has asthma, hay fever and severe intolerance to certain dietary allergens. Yet his skin is fine to the immense delight of his parents. In this case it's likely someone was seeking an obscure reason to explain what the parents now agree was an easily explained mundane protective immune reaction to medicament ingredients in the skin. The boy's eczema was the result of product maintained dermatitis and when the products were discontinued the skin healed itself.

Genetic tests are a fairly new science and we need to allow a settling in period. What I believe we need to challenge is the paradigm that someone needs a genetic defect to explain their eczema. When someone stops using troublesome products on their skin and the skin heals itself, it suggests the products were involved in causing the eczema. That sequence can be explained without the need for a genetic test.

If someone's skincare products are inducing inflammation in the skin, it's the use of those products which explains the disease. If the person has an unusual gene code, that is interesting. When the person stops using those products and their skin heals itself, the gene code will remain the same and still be just as interesting. I simply challenge the paradigm that all eczema patients will have a genetic defect.

Other paradigms exist in the complicated field of eczema. However challenging this set of six is sufficient to develop progressive debate.

What advantages arise from such a broad multi-faceted challenge?

Would it be easier to defeat eczema if we knew:

i. the inflammation could be logically explained and ended,

ii. opaque emollients can cause the inflammation,

iii. moisturisers that repel water can increase the inflammation,

iv. using topical steroids to reduce the inflammation is not in the patients' best long-term interest,

v. the atopic march is not inevitable and can be partly reversed, and

vi. eczema can occur regardless of any genetic defects?

Would that help dispel limiting beliefs and help people break through the boundaries set by others who say eczema can't be cured? Would it help eczema sufferers to progress on their path to a time after eczema? Would it improve their confidence and propel them to becoming an EXeczema® success?

It would, wouldn't it?

EXeczema® Success

Benjamin goes at his own pace!

I had known Dr Harley for years through his other work in preventing diseases. I mentioned to him that my son Benjamin had eczema and only then did Harley tell me of his work on that condition. We had tried lots and lots of different creams from the doctors but nothing seemed to be working and the condition was not getting any better at all.

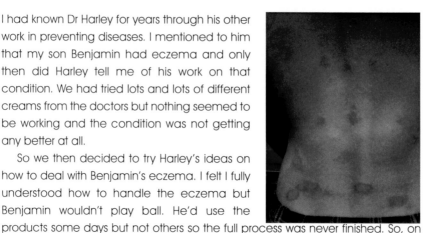

So we then decided to try Harley's ideas on how to deal with Benjamin's eczema. I felt I fully understood how to handle the eczema but Benjamin wouldn't play ball. He'd use the products some days but not others so the full process was never finished. So, on

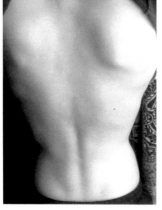

having a conversation with Harley he suggested that we direct it to Benjamin himself and not go via his mum! Harley and I decided the trick would be for Harley to seek Benjamin's views man-to-man. That worked and at last Benjamin kept using the products until his skin healed and the eczema was gone.

Having compared this process with all the products Benjamin had from the doctors, this was amazing and a more natural way of dealing with it.

I have passed on my enthusiasm to other people whose family and friends have also been suffering with eczema, some for a very long time, and they too are now seeing the same amazing results. I will continue to recommend Harley as I feel his work is fantastic and the job he does to help other people deal with this really needs to be heard.

In Benjamin's words,

"It helped me get rid of my eczema really fast and effectively and it has stayed away. Nobody makes comments about my skin when I go swimming now."

Fiona Unick-Wagg
Norfolk

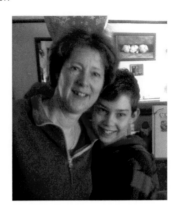

ECZEMA MAY BE MAINTAINED BY BIOMEDICAL TREATMENT: A REVIEW

Abstract

Eczema has a global prevalence. This paper presents the current Biomedical view of its pathogenesis with a brief discussion on how that relates to the traditional Chinese and Indian systems of medicine. Recent advances in Biomedicine demonstrate how biomedical treatments used to manage eczema may help to understand the etiopathogenesis.

Research and best clinical practice have evolved to the point where the skin inflammation which characterizes eczema needs to be combated and overcome. Some of that research is now centred on the very earliest changes which subsequently develop into clinical eczema. It shows the inflammation is in part immune-surveillance suggesting a positive and desirable role in defending the patient. Through several pathways there is a reduction in ceramide and filaggrin-derived amino acids, key components of the epidermal barrier, allowing easy penetration through the defective skin barrier by irritants and allergens. Some of the irritants are applied as medicaments which is designated *product maintained dermatitis*, the author's concern and field of study. Integrative Medicine benefits from combining biomedicine's explanation of the pathophysiology of eczema with the older forms of medicine and great opportunities remain to identify complementary interventions which justify research.

Introduction

Eczema is a skin disease typified by prolonged recurring bouts of skin inflammation (1) with pronounced itching (2), usually with cycles of varying severity (3). While it has been divided into numerous sub-types, in this article it will be considered as one disease with variations. The names Atopic Eczema (AE) and eczema will be used interchangeably here as generic terms.

The incidence of AE has increased in many countries in recent decades (4) with the current accumulative prevalence for children being at about 20% (5). The countries with the highest incidence tend to be the ones with the most developed systems of modern medicine and the cleanest environments, hence an hypothesis that better hygiene and control of hookworm infection explains its higher prevalence (6).

The 1-year prevalence of AE in Danish adults was found to be 14.3% in adults aged 30 to 89 years (7). They reported the prevalence of AE was highest in the younger age groups with a maximum value of 19.2% in those aged 30-40. In all age groups, except those aged 70-90, the prevalence of AE was higher in women compared with men. The association between prevalence and age was statistically significant for all participants as well as each gender group, showing decreasing prevalence with increasing age.

AE adversely affects many aspects of life (8). Sleep disturbance affects up to 60% of children with AE, increasing to 83% during periods of exacerbation (9) and girls, but not boys, report self-perceived impaired health as a result of eczema (10). Among sufferers in their late adolescence, the adverse psychological effect extends to an increased incidence of suicidal thoughts (11).

Early and proactive management could improve the outcome and quality of life for patients (12). As experienced in Australia, managing the disease in infants and young children takes a great deal of family time with an estimated annual cost of 1,142 Australian dollars per child with mild eczema and 6,099 Australian dollars per child with severe eczema (13). AE should not be regarded as a minor skin disorder but as a condition which has the potential to be a major handicap with considerable personal, social and financial consequences both to the family and the community (14).

AE is a comparatively new disease having become prominent in the latter half of last century. Something early in life seems to have caused an imbalance leading to inflammation in the skin. It has been suggested (15) that genes appear to determine an infant's predisposition to AE, but the presence or absence of critical environmental factors probably determines whether or not the disease occurs. This is supported by the observation that AE is more prevalent in first generation infants born in developed countries than in their parents' generation (16). A child's chances of developing AE in the first 6 months of life increased if the mother had eczema and there was an increased incidence of developing AE between 12 and 18 months of age if the child had been treated with antibiotics (55). The advent of modern genetic tests allows much emphasis to be correctly placed on genetics (17) yet the human genome will have changed little in the last 50 years during the pronounced rise in AE incidence. The absence of those genetic differences in most AE patients (18) suggests the genetic changes should be kept in perspective.

The word Atopic in this context denotes an unusual, unexpected or out of place reaction or inflammation with asthma and hay fever (Atopic Rhinitis) being treated with the same therapeutic approach. The three diseases eczema, asthma and hay fever are collectively known as atopic diseases and a patient suffering from any of them is said to be atopic. The phrase 'Atopic March' was introduced to describe the tendency for patients with one of these atopic diseases to subsequently develop one or both of the others (19). The likelihood that AE could lead to the other atopic diseases (20) gives AE increased clinical relevance for patients and financial relevance to the overall healthcare system. AE, occurring often in the first year of life, tends to be the first of the three to be diagnosed, so preventing AE should deliver long-term health and financial benefits (12).

The skin of atopic patients presents challenges for those attempting to ascertain which allergens or irritants induce reaction by the patient's immune system. In 1989 Sonnex and Ryan (21) showed that applying a compound to skin increased the numbers and intensity of subsequent patch test reactions while irritant reactions were not affected.

The search for the initiating factor in the eczema sequence should therefore be conducted well before the clinical disease. The disease has been managed for decades yet it remains common, suggesting that managing the disease is distinct from ending the disease.

The pathogenesis of eczema: the biomedical viewpoint

The pathogenesis of eczema remains poorly understood (22 , 23). Inflammation is a universal feature of eczema and recent articles describe detailed cytokine and chemokine components of the dermatitis (24). Intense pruritis can result from highly active chemicals released into the skin by inflammation and scratching the itch can increase the inflammation worsening the eczema (24). This is a long-held viewpoint dating from at least 1964 (25).

The concept of intrinsic and extrinsic eczema was introduced to distinguish between the two main inflammatory pathways in eczema although now they tend to be seen as sequences in the one disease (26 , 12). The intrinsic mechanism relates to the suboptimal skin barrier resulting in a locally orchestrated immune reaction to penetrating chemicals, typified by a foreign body irritant response. It has recently been shown (15) that anionic surfactants in skincare products cause histidine in corneocytes to be converted to histamine via the enzymic L-histadine decarboxylase pathway in the epidermis. Those epithelial cells lack storage organelles so the histamine is automatically released into the epidermis. This source of histamine is distinct from the histamine stored in, and released from, mast cells in the dermis (27). The clinical features of intrinsic eczema include a relatively milder severity and more intact skin barrier function than for extrinsic eczema (3).

The extrinsic component happens when haptens of less than 500 Daltons in size penetrate the suboptimal skin barrier and become conjugated to the outer membranes of Langerhans cells in the mid to lower epidermis (28). Those Langerhans cells migrate to lymph nodes where T-helper type 2 (Th-2) lymphocytes are cloned into two groups; effector and suppressor. Those cloned T lymphocytes relocate to the immune-surveillance organs, including the skin, and react when their specific allergen next penetrates the skin. If the suppressor Th-2 lymphocytes predominate, there is no inflammatory response when the specific allergen is next encountered and the person is said to be tolerant. When the effector Th-2 lymphocytes predominate, the reaction is the classical IgE-mediated immunological response involving the release of histamine from mast cells. Sensitization is more easily induced when the skin barrier is compromised (28).

Lymphocytes of the same specific clone also localize in the mucosa of other immune-surveillance regions like the nasal turbinates and bronchioles (28). This is believed to explain the "Atopic March" (29). When the specific allergen is encountered in those sites, the classical atopic responses of allergic rhinitis and asthma result if the effector Th-2 lymphocytes predominate (28). Specific skin-derived immune-related molecules are involved in both severe eczema and asthma suggesting a common factor between the diseases (30).

Bacterial involvement complicates eczema with Th-2 cytokines increasing the lethal effect of *Staphylococcus aureus* alpha toxin on less differentiated keratinocytes (31). In acute eczema there is a greater expression of the IL-13 Th-2 cytokines (32) which inhibit keratinocyte differentiation and thereby reduce expression of the filaggrin gene, which is now the focus of research into the pathogenesis of AE (33) and is discussed below. Th-2 cytokines also inhibit the production of lamellar bodies, organelles critical for epidermal barrier formation (31) and inhibit the generation of ceramides (34), the hydrophobic lipids critical for epidermal function.

Eczema patients with IgE sensitization to several microbial antigens had more severe disease facilitating microbial colonization of the skin, resulting in higher frequencies of infection, aggravation of skin inflammation, and more pronounced impairment of the skin barrier (35).

Microorganisms, including *Staphylococcus aureus*, were isolated from 63% of the jars and tubes of skincare products selected from patients. The majority of the microorganisms were isolated from the opening of the tubes or edge of the jars of products, indicating the contaminants were from the users and not intrinsic to the products (36).

The filaggrin gene

In the chemically active epidermal cells of the *stratum granulosum*, expression of the filaggrin gene results in granular deposits of profilaggrin, a large, insoluble polyprotein (4). Each inactive profilaggrin molecule is dephosphorylated and cleaved into filaggrin protein monomers. Filaggrin plays a key role in epidermal barrier function; it aggregates and aligns keratin bundles in the cornified cell envelope (4) and is further degraded to release hygroscopic amino acids with filaggrin being the major source of histidine, urocanic acid and pyrrolidone carboxylic acid (18). In combination with lipids, they become the natural moisturizing factor which forms the intracellular and intercellular layer called the skin barrier.

The skin barrier is mainly localized in the lower *stratum corneum* and is maintained by corneocytes in a lipid-enriched intercellular domain. The intercellular lipid bilayers are formed during the extrusion of the epidermal lamellar body into the transition zone between the *stratum granulosum* and *stratum corneum* (22).

The skin barrier regulates the rate of water loss from the skin (37). Anything which decreases the amount of natural moisturising factor will lead to suboptimal water control by the skin barrier and increased transepidermal water loss and a sensation of xerosis, more commonly known as skin dryness. Dry skin is flaky and rough, exhibits a loss in elasticity, may be pruritic, and has an unsightly appearance (38).

A physical feature of xerosis is fine cracks in the skin (39) which can penetrate deep into the epidermis. Dry skin is characterized by reduced water content in the *stratum corneum*. A healthy *stratum corneum* contains from 15% to 25% water at the skin surface to about 40% at the border between the *stratum corneum* and *stratum granulosum* (40). Scaling on the skin surface becomes visible and pruritis occurs when the relative humidity falls below 10% (41). The feeling of dryness can lead to scratching and further physical damage to the epidermis. All that can happen before erythema or inflammation are visible (39).

Normal skin cleansing with products containing surfactants can be associated with damage to the *stratum corneum* lipids because the surfactants, in addition to providing the desired effect of solubilizing and facilitating the removal of sebum and skin soils, have a propensity to disrupt bilayer lipids by extracting endogenous skin lipids or intercalating into the bilayer (42). Emulsifiers play a key role in this reduction in skin lipid and no emollient product containing sodium lauryl sulfate as a leave-on or washing product should be used by any patient with dry skin (43).

Interleukin-22, a cytokine found within inflamed skin, leads to an inflammatory driven down-regulation of expression of the filaggrin gene (41). IL-17A down-regulates the expression of genes important for cellular adhesion which could affect epidermal barrier formation (44). It is suggested that during episodes of primary dermatitis, whether irritant or atopic in nature, an inflammatory driven down-regulation of filaggrin gene expression is likely to result in very low or even absent levels of filaggrin proteins in the skin that will further decrease skin barrier function and increase penetration of foreign chemicals (45). This reduction in filaggrin and natural moisturising factor happens as a result of inflammation.

Another cause for suboptimal skin barrier function is mutations in the filaggrin gene. Various mutations are specific to certain ethnic groups, with distinct profiles seen in the European and Asian populations (46). Any mutations which decrease expression of the filaggrin gene will result in less natural moisturizing factor and a suboptimal skin barrier. Loss-of-function variants within the filaggrin gene increase the risk of eczema (47). It is estimated that half or more of children with moderate to severe eczema carry filaggrin gene mutations (47). Individuals carrying homozygous null mutations in the filaggrin gene have a complete absence of granules in the epidermal *stratum granulosum* layer (48). Filaggrin deficiency in one in ten Europeans, or complete absence of filaggrin in one in 400, lead to varying degrees of impaired keratinocyte differentiation and barrier function allowing increased transepidermal water loss and, importantly, increased entry of allergens, antigens, and irritant chemicals from the environment (47). Thus, filaggrin-deficient individuals are chronically exposed to insult through the epidermis, which in many cases leads to inflammation of the skin which is eczema (47).

Filaggrin gene demonstrates intragenic copy number variation with alleles encoding 10, 11 or 12 filaggrin monomers; hence, copy number variation may affect the amount of filaggrin expressed in the epidermis (49). A lower number of repeats leads to less profilaggrin being produced and subsequently less natural moisturizing factor.

In spite of this high prevalence of filaggrin gene mutations, it is important to appreciate that reduced natural moisturizing factor and suboptimal skin barrier function occur in people with fully functional filaggrin genes (39). That emphasizes why the gene mutations, important as they are for the individuals concerned, should be kept in perspective in relation to the reductions in natural moisturizing factor which occur in anyone as a result of skin inflammation (18).

Decreased epidermal enzyme activity in lesional and non-lesional skin correlated with reduced *stratum corneum* ceramide content and disturbed skin barrier function (22). The enzyme activity was reduced in non-lesional skin and more significantly reduced in lesional skin, correlating with impaired expression of cornified envelope proteins and keratins, important for skin barrier function. A defective permeability barrier leads to the penetration of environmental allergens into the skin and initiates immunological reactions and inflammation crucially involved in the pathogenesis of eczema (22). Other genetic factors also play a part. The claudin-1 gene plays a critical role in human tight junction function and keratinocyte proliferation (50). Expression of claudin-1 is significantly reduced in non-lesional skin of patients with eczema compared with non-atopic subjects.

Management of Eczema

In spite of the above advances, the pathogenesis of eczema remains largely unknown (23) and not surprisingly there are widely varying treatment strategies including Chinese, Indian, allopathic, homeopathic, holistic, minimalistic and others. All have their place in managing eczema. As with any disease, the effectiveness of treatments for eczema relies heavily on the appropriate skills of the people advocating each treatment. It is not just drug discovery and appropriate identification and dosage of medicaments that is needed, but, as well, the prescriber must be adequately skilled.

The vast majority of children diagnosed with AE cease to have the disease by the age of 20. Some people suggest that shows how effective the treatments are at ending eczema yet others continue to suggest eczema cannot be cured.

The patient outcome will vary depending on whether the intention of the therapy is to:

- address symptoms such as sleeplessness, dry skin, inflammation and pruritis or
- end the eczema and prevent its return.

Recurring 'flare-ups' are anticipated with the former and not expected with the latter.

An extensive clinical enquiry into potential causes of the xerosis, pruritis and dermatitis should precede the diagnosis of eczema (8) and therefore any subsequent suggestions for therapies to manage the disease. That investigation should include consideration of potential contact irritants, systemic immune reactions to factors like food which present as skin erythema and alternative causes of inflamed skin.

Once AE is diagnosed, suggestions on support are available in UK guidance (United Kingdom National Institute for Health and Clinical Excellence) on how to manage the disease, depending on the levels of severity (8).

Management of Dry Skin

Moisturizers and emollients are used to address the symptom of dry skin. The sensation of dry skin results from the skin's inability to adequately control water loss (51). Increased transepidermal water loss indicates that the skin barrier has suboptimal capacity to control the outward flow of water through the skin. Hydrophobic ingredients often used in moisturizers and emollients are intended to form a waterproof layer (43) on the surface of the skin and trap within the skin water which was leaving the body by transcutaneous evaporation. Humectants which chemically bind water within the skin are also common in moisturizers and emollients.

Biomedical Interventions

Topical steroids of varying strength are used to decrease the inflammation. If the inflammation persists despite topical steroid therapy, topical calcineurin inhibitors (tacrolimus or pimecrolimus) can be used to prevent the Th-2 mediated aspect of the immune reaction. It is common to incorporate the topical immuno-suppressants in oil-based creams and ointments with the expectation that they will help maintain a waterproof barrier to decrease transepidermal water loss. If topical immuno-suppressants fail to control the inflammation, systemic cyclosporin can be prescribed by those with the appropriate specialist training (8).

Pruritis can lead to scratching and physical trauma that enhances the inflammation. Cytokines and chemokines generated as part of the inflammatory process can be intensely pruritic (24), further justifying the need to suppress the immune reaction. Specialized clothing, especially night clothing, can reduce the irritation caused by bedding on inflamed skin. Antipruritic therapies, including repeated cooling of inflamed areas have long been well documented (25) and psychological methods intended to reduce the desire to scratch aim to reduce the self-trauma which can result from scratching. Antihistamines have been extensively used to manage the pruritis although it is now suggested that oral antihistamines should not be used routinely in the management of AE in children except for short periods during acute flares to assist with sleep.

When scratching goes deep enough to induce bleeding, bacteria have an increased chance of penetrating the skin resulting in septicemia. Topical antibacterial therapy can be used to decrease the number of bacteria on the skin and intensive systemic antibiotic therapy is required for septicemia.

Scratching, especially unconscious nocturnal scratching by children, can be addressed by occlusive methods, the simplest being to cover finger tips with gloves. Covering inflamed areas of skin with bandages prevents the fingertips reaching the skin. Wet-wrapping involves two layers of bandages or clothing, one moist beneath a dry covering. It is an intervention which requires appropriate training. Emollient may be applied to the skin before the bandages are applied. Occlusive dressing should not be used over infected skin.

Treatment with UV light may be utilised for cases of non-responding severe eczema. Patients are advised to apply sunscreen prior to the treatment to best protect their already damaged skin.

Those guidelines for management of AE in children evolved through best practice supported by evidence-based research (8). The disease symptoms are adequately controlled and while this regime has been in place, 80% of children have consistently grown out of their eczema by the age of twenty. Those children tend to be the ones who do not have recurring flare-ups and they cease to be classed as eczema sufferers. Their eczema is ended and it does not return.

Consideration

Did all those children end their eczema *because* of the biomedical symptom-managing regime? Is it possible that some of the children ended their eczema *despite* the established guidelines? What maintains the eczema in the large group of 20% who do not end their eczema by the age of 20? There are no answers to those questions in the peer-reviewed literature. It may be impossible to determine whether the symptom-managing regime was the primary cause of the 80% ending their eczema, whereas it is very apparent that the regime did not end the eczema for the remaining 20% whose eczema continued.

The concept of managing eczema implies ongoing disease rather than an end of the disease. If it was possible to deliberately end eczema, it could be argued that the words 'end' and 'cure' would be more prominent in the eczema literature. Is there evidence in the peer-reviewed literature which might justify the thought that to 'manage' eczema is to 'maintain' eczema? If so, is AE iatrogenic? Those questions have been posed in a peer-reviewed article (52).

Research opportunities exist in determining what causes the first reduction in natural moisturizing factor which the author believes is the prelude to the entire eczema process.

When the recent peer-reviewed literature is considered, the following sequence of events can be proposed as a pathogenesis for atopic eczema. It is centred on two self-perpetuating and mutually-enhancing cycles of inflammation in the skin as shown in Figure 1.

When the natural moisturizing factor has been depleted to the level where the skin barrier cannot adequately regulate the exit rate of water, the skin barrier also has a suboptimal ability to prevent the entry rate of external chemicals. Moncrieff *et al* (43) suggest the objective of emollient therapy is to correct some of the factors that contribute to dry skin, to restore the skin barrier, and to reduce the likelihood of further damage. Many of the emollient products currently advocated for use on eczematous skin (43) contain high

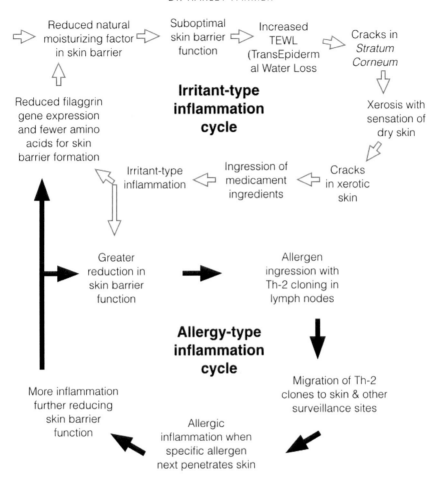

Figure 1. Proposed pathogenesis of Atopic Eczema.

levels of ingredients that are foreign to the human body. They are therefore capable of inducing inflammation when they enter the skin to a depth when they are detected by the immune system. One such ingredient is mineral oil in its various forms and mineral oil is undeniably foreign to the human body. When products containing mineral oil are applied to areas of skin with a suboptimal skin barrier, medicament ingredients can enter the skin and provoke intense inflammation in their own right. That initiates Product Maintained

Dermatitis, a term the author created to indicate how the medicament ingredients which gain entry through the suboptimal skin barrier provoke inflammation as a protective reaction (52). That inflammation, whatever the level of intensity, is the proper and desired protective response to the foreign chemicals which have entered the skin. The level of intensity of the inflammation will be proportionate to the level of foreign chemical ingression.

For many decades it has been common biomedical practice to manage xerosis and eczema with products that are intended to form a superficial hydrophobic layer so no water can pass out, trapping water in the epidermis in order to moisturize the skin (43). For the hydrophobic layer to be achieved, the hydrophobic ingredients within the medicaments must stay on the outer surface of the treated skin.

In fact it has been known since 1992 that petrochemicals permeate throughout the *stratum corneum* interstices (59) leading to petrolatum-induced cleft formation within the intercellular lamellar bilayers. The clefts induce the formation of progressively larger lacunae within the membrane bilayers. Petrolatum caused expansion of intercellular domains, permeating to as low as one layer above the *stratum granulosum-stratum corneum* interface. These observations confirm that petrolatum reaches all levels of the *stratum corneum* and that petrolatum penetrates through the *stratum corneum* via intercellular domains (59).

In addition, recent evidence shows that xerosis is preceded by, and associated with, cracks in the epidermis (39). Those cracks allow ingredients from topical medicaments to pass through the defective skin barrier leading to an inflammatory response against the foreign chemicals. That inflammation will decrease the levels of natural moisturizing factor (45) reducing the effectiveness of the skin barrier leading to increased water loss through the skin. The very products that were applied with the intention of reducing the loss of water through the skin can induce increased epidermal water loss by initiating inflammation which leads to a less optimal skin barrier (52). When that occurs, the use of such hydrophobic topical products to manage dry skin and eczema could harm the patient.

In order to establish which topical products are safe to use on xerotic or eczematous skin, it pays to determine how the skin reacts to individual products. The reactions can be patient specific and vary depending on whether a specific patch of skin has suboptimal skin barrier function. If inflammation occurs following the application of products, the products should be deemed capable of inducing and/or maintaining product maintained dermatitis. That means they maintain eczema. Further use of those products on xerotic or eczematous patches can harm the patient. A good example is Aqueous Cream which was widely used for decades and is no longer an appropriate medicament (51).

In contrast, if the sensation of skin dryness ends and the inflammation decreases when specific topical products are applied, those products do not induce product maintained dermatitis and can be used safely on the patient.

On this basis, most of the moisturizers and emollients currently advocated for use on eczema become potentially harmful to patients with eczema. Managing inflamed eczematous skin with products which in themselves induce dermatitis adds to the causes of inflammation for that patient (52).

The same products applied to areas of non-xerotic and non-eczematous skin on the same patient where the skin barrier has optimal capacity are unlikely to be detected by the immune system and will probably not provoke product maintained dermatitis. The products only become potentially harmful when they are applied to areas of skin where the skin barrier is incapable of preventing medicament ingredients penetrating to the depth where they are reacted against by the immune system (52). Applying those products to suboptimal skin maintains the eczema, reinforcing the concept that eczema is what the patient does rather than what the patient has (25).

The level of inflammation in eczematous skin tends to be proportionate to the level of injurious challenges. Eczematous inflammation is an indication of how much protection the immune system has been provoked into providing in order to protect the patient. The inflammatory reaction is appropriate and correct and does not indicate something is wrong with the immune system (25 , 52). It is what should be hoped for when chemicals which provoke the immune system into inflammation penetrate the defective skin barrier and are detected by the immune system.

Using immune-modulating therapies to reduce this protective inflammation *without* simultaneously removing the injurious challenges increases the danger to the patient and becomes contra-indicated. Such an action would constitute iatrogenic maintenance of the eczema (52). It is correct to address the inflammation but not in the absence of a credible effort to address the cause of the inflammation. By way of example, it is appropriate to advocate the application of topical steroids or calcineurin inhibitors in order to control the injurious inflammation, but if those anti-inflammatory drugs are carried in medicaments containing mineral oil, the latter could be causing the inflammation the drugs are intended to eliminate.

Long-term use of topical corticosteroids leads to depletion of s*tratum corneum* intercellular lipid lamellae and barrier function abnormalities (56) suggesting the diminution of the s*tratum corneum* intercellular lipid lamellae playing an important part in the pathogenesis of barrier disfunction. Furthermore, short-term glucocorticoid use inhibits epidermal lipid synthesis, resulting in a decrease in lipid precursors available for the formation of lamellar bodies and the downstream generation of lamellar bilayers, which mediate permeability barrier function (57) .

Even the stress of taking examinations led to stress-induced derangements in epidermal function and the subjects who demonstrated the greatest increase in perceived psychologic stress also displayed the greatest abnormality in barrier recovery rates considered to be relevant as precipitators of inflammatory dermatoses (58).

Severe AE where the patient is scratching to the point of allowing entry of bacteria into the circulation must be treated in an aggressive manner (8). That is likely to require the use of immune suppressing drugs until the threat of bacterial ingression as a result of injurious scratching is overcome. Once the severity of the eczema is adequately reduced, the use of immune suppressants ceases to be so appropriate. That is an excellent time to investigate whether any of the ingredients in topical products suggested for use on eczema will in themselves induce inflammation when they penetrate the weakened skin barrier. If any of the ingredients have that propensity, the use of products containing them becomes contra-indicated because of the likelihood of iatrogenic product maintained dermatitis (52).

Complementary and Alternative Medicine

Anxious parents faced with a very unhappy child will often turn to Complementary and Alternative Medicine if they have decided hurried biomedical consultations have been of little help. Both Chinese and Indian systems of medicine have been used to treat dermatitis for thousands of years. They emphasize constitutional imbalance and their enquiry into this tends to be lengthy which is in itself therapeutic. The Chinese herbalist chooses several herbs, to make tea, one or two being especially aimed at the problem diagnosed as an imbalance of which both tongue and pulse may provide help with the choice of herb. Other herbs may be enhancing of the lead herb or protective against known adverse reactions. Compared to biomedicine the dose is vague and can be altered according to response.

In the Indian Ayurveda form of medicine the approach is to improve digestion, provide a whole body oil massage, encourage whole body sweating and to purge. Counselling and yoga relaxation exercises are added (53). The Foundation for Revitalization of Local Health Traditions based in Bangalore has developed multidisciplinary computerized databases on medicinal plants. It believes in the principal that the natural product containing many chemicals in balance is safer than a single isolated extract.

Biomedicine was also once more concerned with digestion and gastrointestinal allergy. As early as 1936, it was advocated that cow milk be replaced by goat milk and milk substitutes. Eventually doubts about the effectiveness of these regimens, as well as their safety, led to an editorial in the British Medical Journal which dampened enthusiasm for the substitutes to breast milk (15). In some parts of India where the environment is often heavily contaminated with faeces, breast feeding should be encouraged and anxiety assuaged by prolonged consultation.

This review is intended to demonstrate how biomedicine's sometimes overzealous use of modern manmade chemicals in topical skincare products can cause and then maintain eczema, a modern form of dermatitis. The incidence of eczema has significantly increased around the world in recent decades regardless of whether the local prevailing system of medicine was the newer biomedicine or the older Chinese and Indian systems. That suggested something new might be happening which induced the author to seek modern clues, a search that resulted in this review.

Very recent revelations in the biomedical literature show there are two basic ways to reduce the functionality of the skin barrier. The first is with high detergent/emulsifier activity in topical products which extract lipid from the skin barrier. The other is any form of inflammation within the skin as that reduces the amount of filaggrin-derived amino acids available to form the natural moisturising factor within the skin barrier.

A modern phenomenon of the last half century is topical cosmetic skincare products that combine manmade chemicals that have strong detergent activity with purified mineral oils. It has recently been shown how the former can weaken the skin barrier by depleting ceramides allowing the mineral oils to enter inducing irritant-type inflammation. In biomedicine, products containing the same two types of purified ingredients are then applied to the eczematous skin as a treatment.

The older systems of medicine would not advocate applying more of the products which caused a disease condition. Nor should they be expected to have answers for what is a modern concept of causing an imbalance with a type of product and then using the same type of product to treat the imbalance. AE demonstrates how biomedicine can sometimes focus on the use of purified manmade chemicals to the detriment of patients. When an imbalance is treated with the cause of that imbalance, no system of medicine, ancient or modern, can be expected to correct the imbalance until the cause is removed.

It is hoped this review will lead to AE patients being directed to other types of topical skincare products which do not damage the skin barrier or induce skin inflammation. This will become increasingly relevant around the world as multinational branded skincare products containing both detergents and mineral oils become more widely available for sale.

Modern biomedicine and ancient Chinese and Ayurvedic Indian medicines have many more similarities than differences. All teach that the initial skin dryness and subsequent hyperaemia seen in eczema are an indication of imbalance. The differences emerge in the resources available to those aiming to assist the patient. The older forms of medicine rely on products derived from natural sources, the only ones available in ancient times. Those options will have evolved through some form of trial and error leading, over time, to what are now established practices.

Modern biomedicine has evolved to utilize recently created artificial chemicals like the anionic surfactants found in many topical medicaments. Those new products gave biomedical practitioners new options which justified their use. In a comparatively short time, it became apparent that some of the new products were associated with adverse effects. Aqueous Cream is a recent example; a product based on an anionic surfactant and mineral oil which was heralded as a great advance and is now considered a hazard on skin. Rather than viewing such products as failures, the author suggests they can be seen as part of a useful learning process. Many other skincare products contain surfactant/emulsifier and mineral oils are still being advocated for use on xerotic and eczematous skin. Part of the beneficial learning experience would involve determining which of those products share the same deleterious effects as Aqueous Cream.

Long ago, similar learning experiences would have happened in the progressive development of Chinese and Indian medicines.

The major difference between the older forms of medicine and modern biomedicine is the rate of progress. In just a few generations, the science of biomedicine has provided molecular-level evidence of the biochemical and physiological changes which precede the dry skin leading to AE. That information is of tremendous value to everyone. Like all new knowledge, only time will tell how it should be used to the benefit of mankind.

Integrative Medicine

Integrative Medicine seeks to be inclusive. It allows the utilization of everything that is helpful from all sources. The older Chinese and Ayurvedic medicines bring the advantage of time-honoured learning, while modern biomedicine has made important contributions on how the body works. We have the privileged opportunity to combine ancient knowledge on herbs and minerals with modern artificial chemicals, all within the context of our new knowledge of biochemistry and physiology. A recent example of how the modern science available in biomedicine can assist the ancient forms of medicine arose when it was shown that olive oil was detrimental to human skin (54). It has long been common to massage the skin of infants with plant oils on the presumption that plant oils are safe, yet this recent revelation shows why more research is required to establish which plant oils are beneficial to skin and especially the skin of babies.

As always, the outcome for patients will rest on the skills, knowledge, perspective and training of the person responsible for their care.

References

1. Sher LG, Chang J, Patel IB, Balkrishnan R, Fleischer JR AB. Relieving the pruritis of atopic dermatitis: a meta-analysis. *Acta Derm Venereol* (2012) **92**:455-61.
2. O'Neill JL, Chan YH, Rapp SR, Yosipovitch G. Differences in itch characteristics between psoriasis and atopic dermatitis patients: results of a web-based questionnaire. *Acta Derm Venereol* (2011) **91**:537-540.
3. Tokura Y. Extrinsic and intrinsic types of atopic dermatitis. *J Dermatol Sci* (2010) **58**:1-7.
4. Schultz Larsen F, Hanifin JM. Secular change in the occurrence of atopic dermatitis. *Acta Derm Venereol* (1992) Suppl. **176**:7-12.
5. Olesen AB, Bang K, Juul S, Thestrup-Pedersen K. Stable incidence of atopic dermatitis among children in Denmark during the 1990s. *Acta Derm Venereol* (2005) **85**:244-247.
6. Mpairwe H, Ndibazza J, Webb EL, Nampijja M, Muhangi L, Apule B et al. Maternal hookworm modifies risk factors for childhood eczema: results from a birth cohort in Uganda. *Paediatr Allergy Immunol* (2014) **25**:481-8.
7. Vinding GR, Zarchi K, Ibler KS, Miller IM, Ellervik C, Jemec GBE. Is adult atopic eczema more common than we think? - a population-based study in Danish adults. *Acta Derma Venereol* (2014) **94**:480-2.
8. Carr D, Clark C, Cork MJ, Cox H, Gilmour E, Lancaster W et al. *Atopic Eczema in Children. Management of atopic eczema in children from birth up to the age of 12 years*. London: National Institute for Health and Care Excellence. (2007). http://www.nice.org.uk/guidance/CG57
9. Camfferman D, Kennedy JD, Gold M, Martin AJ, Lushington K. Eczema and sleep and its relationship to daytime functioning in children. *Sleep Med Rev* (2010) **14**:359-369.
10. Ballardini N, Ostblom E, Wahlgren C, Kull I. Mild Eczema Affects Self-perceived Health among Pre-adolescent Girls. *Acta Derm Venereol* (2014) **94**:312-6.

11. Halvorsen AJ, Lien L, Dalgard F, Bjertness E, Stern RS. Suicidal ideation, mental health problems, and social function in adolescents with eczema: a population-based study. *J Invest Dermatol* (2014) **134**:1847-1854.
12. Bieber T. Atopic Dermatitis. *N Eng J Med* (2008) **358**:1483-1494.
13. Kemp AS. Atopic eczema: its social and financial costs. *J Paediatr Child Health* (1999) **35**:229-231.
14. Kemp AS. Cost of illness of atopic dermatitis in children: a societal perspective. *PharmacoEconomics* (2003) **21**:105-13.
15. Atherton DJ. Breast Feeding and atopic eczema, Editorial. *Br Med J* (1983) **287**:775-6.
16. George S, Berth-Jones J, Grahame-Browne RAC. A Possible Explanation for the increased Referral of Atopic Dermatitis from the Asian Community in Leicester. *Br J Dermatol* (1997) **136**:494-7.
17. Irvine AD, McLean WH. Breaking the (un)sound barrier: filaggrin is a major gene for atopic dermatitis. *J Invest Dermatol* (2006) **126**:1200-2.
18. Kezic S, O'Regan GM, Yau N, Sandilands A, Chen H, Campbell LE et al. Level of filaggrin degradation products are influenced by both filaggrin genotype and atopic dermatitis severity. *Allergy* (2011) **66**: 934-940.
19. Burgess JA, Lowe AJ, Matheson MC, Varigos G, Abramson MJ, Dharmage SC. Does eczema lead to asthma? *J Asthma* (2009) **46**:429-436.
20. Jensen J, Weppner M, Dahnhardt-Pfeiffer S, Neumann C, Brautigam M, Schwarz T et al. Effects of Primecrolimus compared to Triamcinolone Acetonide cream on skin barrier structure in atopic dermatitis: a randomized, double-blind, right-left trial. *Acta Derm Venereol* (2013) **93**:515-9.
21. Sonnex TS, Ryan TJ. An investigation of the angry back syndrome using Trafuril. *Br J Dermatol* (1987) **116**:361-370.
22. Jensen JM, Folster-Holst R, Baranowsky A, Schunck M, Winoto-Morbach S, Neumann C et al. Impaired sphingo-myelinase activity and epidermal differentiation in atopic dermatitis. *J Invest Dermatol* (2004) **122**:1423-31.
23. Park SY, Oh S, Kim EJ, Yoon SY, Park HS, Yoon H et al. Utility of eosinophil cationic protein levels in the diagnosis of intrinsic atopic dermatitis. *Acta Derm Venereol* (2014) **94**:333-4.
24. Kimura T, Sugaya M, Suga H, Morimura S, Miyamoto A, Kai H et al. Variations in serum TARC and I-TAC levels reflect minor changes in disease activity and pruritis in atopic dermatitis. *Acta Derm Venereol* (2014) **94**:331-2.
25. Bobroff A. *Eczema. Its nature, cure and prevention.* Charles Thomas Publishing, Springfield, Illinois, USA (1962). 21 p and 30 p.
26. Johansson SGO, Bieber T, Dahl R, Friedmann P, Lanier BQ, Lockey RF et al. Revised nomenclature for allergy for global use: report of the Nomenclature Review Committee of the World Allergy Organization, October 2003. *J Allergy Clin Immunol* (2004) **113**:832-6.
27. Inami Y, Sasaki A, Andoh T, Kuraishi Y. Surfactant-induced chronic pruritis: Role of L-Histidine Decarboxylase expression and histamine production in epidermis. *Acta Derm Venereol* (2014) **94**:645-50.
28. Rietschel RL, Fowler JF. *Fisher's Contact Dermatitis 5th edition* edited by Lippincott Williams & Wilkins, Philadelphia. (2001)
29. Bingefors K, Svensson A, Isacson D, Lindberg M. Self-reported lifetime prevalence of atopic dermatitis and co-morbidity with asthma and eczema in adulthood: A population-based cross-sectional survey. *Acta Derm Venereol* (2013) **93**:438-41.

30. Demehri S, Morimoto M, Holtzman MJ, Kopan R. Skin-Derived TSLP Triggers Progression from Epidermal-Barrier Defects to Asthma. *PLoS Biology* (2009) **7**(5):e1000067.

31. Brauweiler AM, Goleva E, Leung YM. Th2 cytokines increase *Staphylococcus aureus* alpha toxin-induced keratinocyte death through the signal transducer and activator of Transcription 6 (STAT6). *J Invest Dermatol* (2014) **134**:2114-21.

32. Hamid Q, Naseer T, Minshall EM, Song YL, Boguniewicz M, Leung DY. In vivo expression of IL12 and IL-13 in atopic dermatitis. *J Allergy Clin Immunol* (1996) **98**:225-31.

33. Howell MD, Kim BE, Gao P, Grant AV, Boguniewicz M, DeBenedetto A et al. Cytokine modulation of atopic dermatitis filaggrin skin expression. *J Allergy Clin Immunol* (2007) **120**:150-5.

34. Sawada E, Yoshida N, Sugiura A, Imokawa G. Th1 cytokines accentuate but Th2 cytokines attenuate ceramide production in the stratum corneum of human epidermal equivalents: an implication for the disrupted barrier mechanism in atopic dermatitis. *J Dermatol Sci* (2012) **68**:25-35.

35. Sonesson A, Bartosik J, Christiansen J, Roscher I, Nilsson F, Schmidtchen A et al. Sensitization to skin-associated microorganisms in adult patients with atopic dermatitis is of important for disease severity. *Acta Derm Venereol* (2013) **93**:340-5.

36. Lundov MD, Johansen JD, Zachariae C, Moesby L. Creams used by hand eczema patients are often contaminated with *Staphylococcus aureus*. *Acta Derm Venereol* (2012) **92**:441-2.

37. Cork MJ, Danby SG, Vasilopoulos Y, Hadgraft J, Lane ME, Mustafa M et al. Epidermal barrier dysfunction in atopic dermatitis. *J Invest Dermatol* (2009) **129**:1892-908.

38. Proksch E, Lachapelle JM. The management of dry skin with topical emollients - recent perspectives. *J Dtsch Dermatol Ges* (2005) **3**:768-74.

39. Thyssen JP, Johansen JD, Zachariae C, Menne T, Linneberg A. Xerosis is associated with atopic dermatitis, hand eczema and contact sensitization independent to filaggrin gene mutation. *Acta Derm Venereol* (2013a) **93**:406-10.

40. Caspers PJ, Lucassen GW, Carter EA, Bruining HA, Puppels GJ. *In vivo* confocal Raman microspectroscopy of the skin: noninvasive determination of molecular concentration profiles. *J Invest Dermatol* (2001) **116**:434-42.

41. Gutowska-Owsiak D, Schaupp AL, Salimi M, Taylor S, Off GS. Interleukin-22 downregulates filaggrin expression and affects expression of profilaggrin processing enzymes. *Br J Dermatol* (2011) **165**:492-8.

42. Ananthapadmanabhan KP, Mukherjee S, Chandar P. Stratum corneum fatty acids: their critical role in preserving barrier integrity during cleansing. *Int J Cos Sci* (2013) **35**:337-45.

43. Moncrieff G, Cork M, Lawton S, Kokiet S, Daly C, Clark C. Use of emollients in dry-skin conditions: consensus statement. *Clin Exp Dermatol* (2013) **3**:231-8.

44. Gutowska-Owsiak D, Schaupp AL, Salimi M, Selvakumar TA, McPherson T, Taylor S et al. IL-17 downregulates filaggrin and affects keratinocyte expression of genes associated with cellular adhesion. *Exp Dermatol* (2012) **21**:104-10.

45. Thyssen JP, Linneberg A, Ross-Hansen K, Carlsen BC, Meldgaard M, Szecsi PB et al. Filaggrin mutations are strongly associated with contact sensitization in individuals with dermatitis. *Contact Dermatitis* (2013b) **68**:273-6.

46. Chen H, Common JE, Haines RL, Balakrishnan A, Brown SJ, Goh CSM et al. Wide spectrum of filaggrin-null mutations in atopic dermatitis highlight

differences between Singaporean Chinese and European populations. *Br J Dermatol* (2011) **165**:106-24.

47. Irvine AD, McLean WH, Leung DY. Filaggrin mutations associated with skin and allergic diseases. *N Eng J Med* (2011) **365**:1315-27.

48. Smith FJ, Irvine AD, Terron-Kwiatkowski A, Sandilands A, Campbell LE, Zhao Y et al. Loss-of-function mutations in the gene encoding filaggrin cause ichthyosis vulgaris. *Nat Genet* (2006) **38**:337-42.

49. Brown SJ, Kroboth K, Sandilands A, Campbell LE, Pohler E, Kezic S et al. Intragenic copy number variation within filaggrin contributes to the risk of atopic dermatitis with a dose-dependent effect. *J Invest Dermatol* (2012) **132**: 98-104.

50. De DA, Rafaels NM, McGirt LY, Ivanov AI, Georas SN, Cheadle C et al. Tight junction defects in patients with atopic dermatitis. *J Allergy Clin Immunol* (2011) **127**:773-86.

51. Cork MJ, Timmins I, Holden C, Holden C, Carr J, Berry V et al. An audit of adverse drug reactions to aqueous cream in children with atopic eczema. *Pharmaceut J* (2003) **271**: 746-7.

52. Farmer H. Is atopic eczema iatrogenic? *J Alt Comp Med* (2013) **19**:681-3.

53. Hegde P, Hemanth DT, Emmi SV, Shilpa MP, Shindhe PS, Santosh YM. A case discussion on eczema. *Int J Ayurveda Res* (2010) **1**:268-70.

54. Danby SG, AlEnezi T, Sultan A, Lavender T, Chittock J, Brown, K, et al. Effect of olive and sunflower seed oil on the adult skin barrier: implications for neonatal skin care. *Pediatr Dermatol* (2013) **30**:42–50.

55. Loo EXL, Shek LP, Goh A, Teoh OH, Chan YH, Soh SE, Saw SM, Kwek K, Gluckman PD, Godfrey KM, Chong YS, Lee BW, Van Bever HP. Atopic Dermatitis in Early Life: Evidence for at Least Three Phenotypes? Results from the GUSTO Study. *Int Arch Allergy Immunol* (2015) **166**: 273-279.

56. Sheu HM, Lee JYY, Chai CY, Kuo KW. Depletion of stratum corneum intercellular lipid lamellae and barrier function abnormalities after long-term topical corticosteroid. *Br J Dermatol* (1997) **136**: 884-890.

57. Kao JS, Fluhr JW, Man MQ, Fowler AJ, Hachem JP, Crumrine D, Ahn SU, Brown BE, Elias PM, Feingold KR. Short-term glucocorticoid treatment compromises both permeability barrier homeostasis and stratum corneum integrity: inhibition of epidermal lipid synthesis accounts for functional abnormalities. *J Invest Dermatol* (2003) **120**: 456-464.

58. Garg A, Chren MM, Sands LP, Matsui MS, Marenus KD, Feingold KR, Elias PM. Psychological stress perturbs epidermal permeability barrier homeostasis: implications for the pathogenesis of stress-associated skin disorders. *Arch Dermatol (*20010 **137**: 53-59.

59. Ghadially R, Lalkier-Sorensen L, Elias PM. Effects of petrolatum on stratum corneum structure and function. *J Am Acad Dermatol* (1992) **26**: 387-396.